Critical Events in Anesthesia

A Clinical Guide for Nurse Anesthetists

Sass Elisha

Mark Gabot

Jeremy Heiner

Published by
American Association of Nurse Anesthetists

Authors

Sass Elisha, CRNA, EdD
Assistant Director
Kaiser Permanente School of Anesthesia
California State University Fullerton

Mark Gabot, CRNA, MSN
Academic and Clinical Educator
Kaiser Permanente School of Anesthesia
California State University Fullerton

Jeremy Heiner, CRNA, MSN
Academic and Clinical Educator
Kaiser Permanente School of Anesthesia
California State University Fullerton

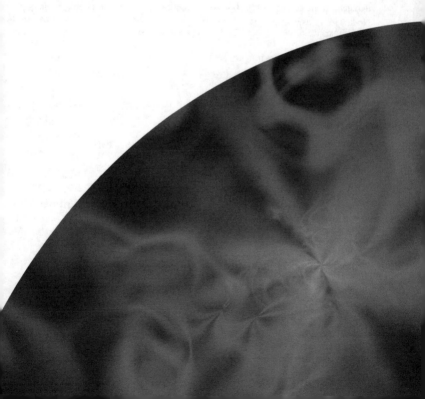

American Association of Nurse Anesthetists
222 South Prospect Avenue
Park Ridge, IL 60068-4001

Printed in the United States of America

Last digit indicates print number: 10 9 8 7 6 5 4 3 2 1

The author(s) and publisher have done everything possible to make this book accurate, up to date, and in accord with accepted standards at the time of publication. The authors, editors, and publisher are not responsible for errors or omissions or for consequences from application of the book, and make no warranty, expressed or implied, in regard to the contents of the book. Any practice described in this book should be applied by the reader in accordance with professional standards of care used in regard to the unique circumstances that may apply in each situation.

Library of Congress Cataloging-in-Publication Data

Elisha, Sass.
  Critical events in anesthesia : a clinical guide for nurse anesthetists / Sass Elisha, Mark Gabot, Jeremy Heiner.
    p. ; cm.
  Includes bibliographical references and index.
  ISBN 978-0-9700279-9-3 (alk. paper)
  I. Gabot, Mark. II. Heiner, Jeremy. III. American Association of Nurse Anesthetists. IV. Title.
  [DNLM: 1. Anesthesia--adverse effects--Handbooks. 2. Anesthesia--nursing--Handbooks.
3. Intraoperative Complications--nursing--Handbooks. 4. Nurse Anesthetists--Handbooks.
5. Perioperative Nursing--methods--Handbooks. WY 49]

  617.9'6--dc23
                        2012021289

Foreword

As healthcare in the United States continues to evolve, Certified Registered Nurse Anesthetists (CRNAs) will remain essential contributors in providing high-quality care. CRNAs have been at the forefront of the remarkable advances in anesthesia clinical practice. The increased incidence and complexity of comorbid diseases that develop during surgery and anesthesia make it essential that all anesthesia providers are able to recognize, prevent when possible, diagnose, and rapidly treat anesthetic complications and emergencies. Methodological and proactive approaches to crisis management are core concepts to help ensure patient safety. Technical, cognitive, and psychomotor performance, as well as effective communication within a team environment, is facilitated by applying the principles contained in this innovative new book.

The information has been written in an easy-to-read, uniform, and concise format so *Critical Events in Anesthesia* will be a valuable resource for practicing clinicians, educators, and students. The content presented makes this text an ideal reference for educators to use during simulation and academic instruction. In addition, it is a practical resource for novice and advanced learners to improve recognition, clinical decision making, and treatment of anesthetic complications. Common major critical events are presented, which makes this text an ideal companion as a quick reference for anesthetists in the operating room. The authors of this book incorporate their knowledge from years of clinical practice, education, and anesthesia simulation, making each chapter a vital source for critical event management.

In this age of increased accountability and information access, *Critical Events in Anesthesia* will continue to be a valuable resource for clinical practitioners. I am confident that you will find yourself frequently reviewing the chapter material throughout your career as you continue to acquire knowledge and enhance the practice of anesthesia.

John Nagelhout, CRNA, PhD, FAAN
Director
Kaiser Permanente School of Anesthesia
California State University Fullerton

Preface

Our purpose for writing this text was to assist anesthesia providers in improving their knowledge related to diagnosis and treatment of events that commonly and uncommonly occur during anesthetic management. The topics are presented in a concise format that provides readers with all the necessary information in one resource. It is our distinct hope that the information contained within this book helps improve care that results in superior patient outcomes.

Sass Elisha, CRNA, EdD
Mark Gabot, CRNA, MSN
Jeremy Heiner, CRNA, MSN

Acknowledgments

The authors thank their families, friends, and the others listed below for their continual support throughout this academic endeavor.

Kaiser Permanente
Pasadena, California

Kaiser Permanente School of Anesthesia
California State University Fullerton
Pasadena, California

John Nagelhout, CRNA, PhD, FAAN
Director
Kaiser Permanente School of Anesthesia
California State University Fullerton

Sandy Bordi, CRNA, MSN
Academic and Clinical Educator
Kaiser Permanente School of Anesthesia
California State University Fullerton

Jennifer Thompson, CRNA, MSN
Academic and Clinical Educator
Kaiser Permanente School of Anesthesia
California State University Fullerton

Brandon Gabot
Medical Illustrator

Sally Aquino, BA
Publications Manager and Managing Editor, *AANA Journal*
American Association of Nurse Anesthetists

Jeannene Sarno, BA
Manager, Design/Production
American Association of Nurse Anesthetists

Jean Winkler, BA
Editorial Specialist
American Association of Nurse Anesthetists

Larry Sawyer, BA
Associate Editor
American Association of Nurse Anesthetists

Abbreviations

AAI	Acute adrenal insufficiency
ABG	Arterial blood gas
ACE	Angiotensin-converting enzyme
ACLS	Advanced cardiac life support
ACTH	Adrenocorticotropic hormone
AICD	Automatic implantable cardioverter-defibrillator
APH	Antepartum hemorrhage
ARDS	Acute respiratory distress syndrome
ARF	Acute renal failure
ASA	American Society of Anesthesiologists
ATP	Adenosine triphosphate
AV	Atrioventricular
BiPAP	Biphasic positive airway pressure
BUN	Blood urea nitrogen
CAD	Coronary artery disease
CBC	Complete blood cell
CHF	Congestive heart failure
CK	Creatine kinase
CKD	Chronic kidney disease
CK-MB	Creatine kinase, M and B subunits
CNS	Central nervous system
COPD	Chronic obstructive pulmonary disease
CPAP	Continuous positive airway pressure
CRF	Chronic renal failure
CRMD	Cardiac rhythm management device
CRPS	Complex regional pain syndrome
CSF	Cerebrospinal fluid
CT	Computed tomography
CVP	Central venous pressure
DIC	Disseminated intravascular coagulation
ECG	Electrocardiogram
ED	Emergency department
EMI	Electromagnetic interference
ESRD	End-stage renal disease
$ETCO_2$	End-tidal carbon dioxide
ETT	Endotracheal tube

FFP	Fresh frozen plasma
F_{IO_2}	Fraction of inspired oxygen
GI	Gastrointestinal
HELLP	Hemolysis, elevated liver function, low platelets
HPA	Hypothalamic-pituitary-adrenal
ICU	Intensive care unit
IgE	Immunoglobulin E
INR	International normalized ratio
IPH	Intrapartum hemorrhage
IV	Intravenous
LA	Local anesthetic
LLDP	Left lateral decubitus position
LMA	Laryngeal mask airway
MAP	Mean arterial pressure
MH	Malignant hyperthermia
MRI	Magnetic resonance imaging
NG	Nasogastric
NPO	Nothing by mouth (nil per os)
NSAIDs	Nonsteroidal anti-inflammatory drugs
OR	Operating room
Pa_{CO_2}	Partial pressure of carbon dioxide in arterial blood
PACU	Postanesthesia care unit
PALS	Pediatric advanced life support
Pa_{O_2}	Partial pressure of oxygen in arterial blood
PCWP	Pulmonary capillary wedge pressure
PEEP	Positive end-expiratory pressure
PIP	Peak inspiratory pressure
PPH	Postpartum hemorrhage
PO	By mouth (per os)
PRBC	Packed red blood cells
PT	Prothrombin time
PTT	Partial thromboplastin time
RYR	Ryanodine
SIADH	Syndrome of inappropriate antidiuretic hormone secretion
SNS	Sympathetic nervous system
Sp_{O_2}	Oxygen saturation as measured by pulse oximetry
SQ	Subcutaneous
SVR	Systemic vascular resistance

TIVA	Total intravenous anesthesia
TRALI	Transfusion-related lung injury
TURP	Transurethral resection of the prostrate
VAE	Venous air embolism
WHO	World Health Organization
WPW	Wolff-Parkinson-White (syndrome)

Contents

Chapter 1
Acute Adrenal Crisis

Treatment

- Ventilate or intubate for respiratory distress or arrest.
- Administer hydrocortisone (100 mg) IV bolus, followed by hydrocortisone (50-100 mg) IV every 6 hours for 24 hours.
- Administer an isotonic crystalloid (eg, lactated Ringer's solution or normal saline) to expand intravascular volume.
- Administer $D_{50}W$ IV bolus if hypoglycemia is present.
- Administer vasopressors or positive inotropic medication to treat hypotension.
- Assess the need for invasive monitoring (eg, arterial line and/or central venous line).
- Monitor laboratory values (eg, electrolytes, cortisol, ACTH, and glucose).
- Monitor for sepsis.
- Identify and treat the underlying cause.
- Perform cardiac resuscitation per American Heart Association ACLS or PALS protocol as necessary.

Physiology and Pathophysiology

The adrenal glands are located immediately superior to the kidneys and secrete cortisol. Hormones that are secreted by the adrenal cortex include (1) mineralocorticoids (primarily aldosterone), (2) glucocorticoids (primarily cortisol), and (3) androgens. Glucocorticoids exert a powerful physiologic effect on every body system. Cortisol is responsible for various physiological reactions including (1) maintenance of blood sugar level, (2) maintenance of fluid and electrolyte status, and (3) maintenance of normal vascular tone.

Secretion of cortisol from the adrenal cortex is dependent on the functional integrity of the HPA axis. AAI can be caused by damage (eg, trauma) or pathology (eg, malignancy or autoimmune disease) to the hypothalamus, anterior pituitary, or adrenal cortex. Patients receiving exogenous steroids perioperatively may develop AAI during episodes of physiological stress due to adrenal cortical atrophy. A single induction dose of etomidate can cause adrenal insufficiency for up to 48 hours after administration. This occurs as a result of inhibition of 11 β-hydroxylase, an enzyme necessary for the production of cortisol. In addition, sepsis and emergency procedures, which are associated with a high incidence of infection, can lead to acute AAI. Acute adrenal insufficiency is a rare but life-threatening event that must be diagnosed and treated expeditiously.

Signs and Symptoms

Respiratory
- Distress or arrest

Cardiovascular
- Cardiac arrest
- Severe hypotension, minimally responsive or unresponsive to vasopressor medications

Other Considerations
- Abdominal pain
- Electrolytes (hyperkalemia, hyponatremia)
- Hypoglycemia
- Hypovolemia
- Metabolic acidosis
- Nausea/vomiting

Differential Diagnosis

Cardiovascular
- Hypotension (see Chapter 22)
- Myocardial ischemia or infarction (see Chapter 28)
- Shock states (see Chapter 34)

Endocrine
- Primary adrenal insufficiency
- Secondary adrenal insufficiency (eg, hypothalamic and/or pituitary gland dysfunction)

Pharmacologic
- Abrupt termination of steroid therapy
- Etomidate

Other Considerations
- Anaphylaxis (see Chapter 5)
- Hemorrhage (see Chapter 18)

Suggested Readings

Elisha S, Gabot M, Giron S. Steroids. In: Ouellette RG, Joyce JA, eds. *Pharmacology for Nurse Anesthesiology.* Sudbury, MA: Jones & Bartlett; 2011:303-313.

Grover VK, Babu R, Bedi SPS. Steroid therapy: current indications in practice. *Indian J Anesth.* 2007;51(5):389-393.

Nagelhout J, Elisha S, Waters E. Should I continue or discontinue that medication? *AANA J.* 2009;77(1):59-73.

Treatment

- Turn patient's head.
- Suction gastric contents from oropharynx.
- Apply cricoid pressure to decrease additional gastric aspiration.
- Intubate immediately.
- Suction trachea and bronchi via endotracheal tube before ventilation.
- Apply positive pressure ventilation.
- Titrate F_{IO_2} to $Spo_2 > 90\%$, $Pao_2 > 60$ mm Hg.
- Consider initiating PEEP.
- Prevention:
  - Adhere to current ASA NPO guidelines.
  - Delay diagnostic or nonemergency surgical procedures.
  - Select an alternative to general anesthesia (regional, neuraxial, or monitored anesthesia care-conscious sedation with local anesthesia).
  - Initiate rapid-sequence induction with application of cricoid pressure.
  - Place NG tube and suction before induction of anesthesia.
  - Place NG tube and suction after induction of anesthesia if gastric distention occurs.
  - Suction oropharynx before extubation and deflation of endotracheal tube cuff.

Treatment (continued)

- Pharmacologic prevention:
  - Metoclopramide IV
  - Histamine (H_2) antagonist IV (60-90 minutes before induction of anesthesia)
  - Sodium citrate, PO

Physiology and Pathophysiology

During the induction of anesthesia, the upper and lower esophageal sphincters relax. Gastric aspiration can occur if intragastric pressure exceeds lower esophageal barrier pressure (eg, high ventilating pressures, increased gastric volume, or bowel obstruction).

Acute gastric aspiration can occur at any time throughout the anesthetic course when the patient's laryngeal reflexes are inhibited. Gastric aspirate can migrate into the lungs, causing chemical irritation and/or destruction of pulmonary tissue. Alveolar capillary membrane edema and degeneration, alveolar type II pneumocyte destruction, and microhemorrhaging all result in hypoxia. The earliest and most reliable sign associated with gastric aspiration is hypoxia.

The severity of the signs and symptoms is dependent on the following:

1. volume aspirated
2. pH of aspirate
3. type of aspirate (Solids cause more pulmonary tissue damage than liquids.)
4. patient's physical condition

Acute gastric aspiration can result in aspiration pneumonitis. This pathophysiological process can be divided into 2 phases: (1) direct chemical injury and (2) inflammatory mediator release. Management of this condition includes positive pressure ventilation and is mainly supportive.

Signs and Symptoms

Respiratory
- Dyspnea
- Gastric secretions in oropharynx
- Hypercarbia
- Hypoxia (earliest and most reliable sign)
- Increased PIP
- Infiltrates on chest radiograph
- Rales and/or rhonchi
- Tachypnea
- Wheezing

Cardiovascular
- Hypertension (early sign), hypotension (late sign in severe aspiration)
- Pulmonary hypertension
- Tachycardia

Other
- DIC

Differential Diagnosis

Respiratory
- ARDS
- Bronchospasm (see Chapter 8)
- ETT migration and/or obstruction
- Hypercarbia (see Chapter 19)
- Hypoxia (see Chapter 24)
- Pneumonia
- Pulmonary edema
- Pulmonary embolism (see Chapter 17)
- Upper respiratory tract infection

Cardiovascular
- CHF

Hematologic
- DIC (see Chapter 14)

Other Considerations
- Anaphylaxis (see Chapter 5)

Suggested Readings

El-Orbany M, Connolly LA. Rapid sequence induction and intubation: current controversy. *Anesth Analg.* 2010;110(5):1318-1325.

Fontes ML, Berger JS, Yao FSF. Aspiration pneumonitis and acute respiratory failure. In: Yao FSF, Malhotra V, Fontes ML, eds. *Yao & Artusio's Anesthesiology: Problem-Oriented Patient Management.* 6th ed. Philadelphia, PA: Lippincott Williams & Wilkins; 2008:48-86.

Rieker M. Respiratory anatomy, physiology, pathophysiology, and anesthesia management. In: Nagelhout JJ, Plaus KL, eds. *Nurse Anesthesia.* 4th ed. St Louis, MO: Saunders Elsevier; 2010:560-629.

Strachan P, Solomita M. Aspiration syndromes: pneumonia and pneumonitis: preventive measures are still the best strategy. *J Respir Dis.* 2007;28(9):370-379.

Chapter 3
Airway Fire/Operating Room Fire

Treatment

- Protect patient and contain fire.

Airway Fire
- Call for help.
- Disconnect circuit.
- Discontinue ventilation and oxygen flow.
- Extinguish airway fire with sterile saline or water.
- Remove ETT.
- Verify fire is extinguished.
- Remove surgical sponges, segments of the burned ETT, and/or other debris that may remain in the airway.
- Re-establish a patent airway and resume ventilation.
- Verify degree of injury using fiberoptic bronchoscope.
- Consider IV or inhaled corticosteroids and/or inhaled racemic epinephrine.
- Consult burn specialists for advanced treatment.

Operating Room Fire
- Immediately remove burning drapes or other material from the patient.
- Extinguish fire with carbon dioxide extinguisher, sterile saline, or water.
- Activate the fire alarm and notify surgical team members.
- Call for help.
- If fire engulfs the patient, disconnect breathing circuit, stop flow of oxygen, and begin manual ventilation with bag valve device.
- Verify that the fire is extinguished.

Treatment (continued)

- Remove the patient from the OR and close doors.
- Turn off the gas supply to OR suite.
- Administer TIVA until the surgery can be completed.
- Report all fires that occur within the OR to the hospital's risk management department.

Prevention of Airway Fire

For monitored anesthesia care and general anesthesia:
- Use low F_{IO_2} (maintain air and/or oxygen blend with an F_{IO_2} of 21%-30%).
- Use vented drapes and low oxygen flow rates during sedation if the patient's head is covered and electrocautery is used.
- Cover facial hair or other body hair with water-soluble gel.
- Soak sterile towels with sterile saline or water and place around surgical area.
- Avoid petroleum-based ointments in surgical area (eg, ophthalmic ointment).
- Consider active evacuation of surgical gas and smoke with suction.
- Moisten sponges that are used near ignition sources (especially near the airway).
- Allow sufficient time for flammable skin preparations to dry.

For general anesthesia:
- Use low F_{IO_2} (maintain air and/or oxygen blend with an F_{IO_2} of 21%-30%).
- Reduce gas flow rates.
- Avoid nitrous oxide.
- Use specially manufactured laser ETT.
- Use jet ventilation or intermittent apnea and extubation.

Prevention of Airway Fire (continued)

Methods to help avoid combustion of ignition sources:
- Avoid placing laser or electrocautery pen on patient or surgical drapes.
- Fill ETT cuff with normal saline and dye to visualize cuff rupture.
- Have sterile saline or water available to extinguish fire if it occurs.
- Protect the patient's eyes with wet gauze and laser goggles.
- Display fire precaution signs inside and outside OR.

Physiology and Pathophysiology

Each year an estimated 600 OR fires occur in the United States, and the incidence is increasing. This devastating complication endangers the lives of patients and surgical personnel alike. Because a fire can overcome the entire OR in seconds, it is imperative that all anesthesia providers take measures to decrease the potential for a fire and have a definitive plan if one occurs.

The 3 ingredients necessary to ignite a fire are oxygen, heat, and fuel. The potential for fire within the OR exists because:
1. Supra-atmospheric concentrations of oxygen are frequently administered during anesthesia.
2. Multiple heat and ignition sources are used in the OR (eg, electrocautery, lasers, and numerous electrical devices).
3. Fuel sources are present in the OR and in contact with the staff and patient (surgical towels, sponges, drapes, and gowns).

In addition, when lasers are used for surgical procedures, the concentrated energy may be focused in the airway. The beam may inadvertently penetrate the ETT or ignite drapes, resulting in fire. A list of commonly used lasers is included in Table 3.1.

Physiology and Pathophysiology (continued)

Heat and/or fire can be directed into the lungs, trachea, and upper airway, causing catastrophic tissue damage, airway edema, and death. Specific surgical procedures such as tracheostomy and tracheoesophageal fistula repair can increase the risk of airway fire because of the use of electrocautery within and around the airway and trachea. Anaerobic organisms such as bacteria and peptostreptococci and aerobic organisms such as staphylococci and *Pseudomonas* may be present in patients with lung infections. The gas produced by these bacteria may increase the possibility of airway fires. Taking precautions and preventing an airway and/or OR fire is vital. It is essential for the entire surgical team to work cohesively and formulate a comprehensive plan to protect the patient and OR staff from fire if it occurs.

Table 3.1. Lasers Commonly Used in the Operating Room

Laser	Application (surgical specialty)
Carbon dioxide	General surgery, orthopedics, gynecology, urology, otolaryngology, plastic surgery
Nd:YAG	Gastroenterology, pulmonology, urology, dermatology, ophthalmology
Ho:YAG	Orthopedics, urology
Diode	Dermatology, ophthalmology, otolaryngology, plastic surgery, pain management
Argon	Ophthalmology, otolaryngology, plastic surgery, dermatology, gynecology

Abbreviations: Nd:YAG, neodymium:yttrium-aluminum-garnet; Ho:YAG, holmium:yttrium-aluminum-garnet.

Signs and Symptoms

Respiratory
- Decreased Sp_{O_2}
- Stridor
- Wheezing

Cardiovascular
- Hypertension
- Tachycardia

Other Considerations
- Inability to sustain positive pressure ventilation
- Large cuff leak during manual ventilation
- Loss of $ETCO_2$ waveform

- Machine alarms indicate low tidal volume
- Odor of burning drapes or gauze
- Odor of burning tissue
- Odor of inhalation agent
- Smoke and fire
- Spark, flash, and/or popping sound
- Visual identification of fire
- Visual identification by surgeon of spark, cuff rupture, or fire

Differential Diagnosis

Respiratory
- Bronchospasm (see Chapter 8)
- ETT cuff rupture
- Hypercarbia (see Chapter 19)
- Hypoxia (see Chapter 24)
- Inadvertent ETT removal
- Stridor (see Chapter 35)

Cardiovascular
- Cardiac arrest
- Cardiac dysrhythmias (see Chapter 9)

Other Considerations
- Acidosis
- Circuit disconnect
- Machine failure (see Chapter 6)

Suggested Readings

American Society of Anesthesiologists Task Force on Operating Room Fires, Caplan RA, Barker SJ, et al. Practice advisory for the prevention and management of operating room fires. *Anesthesiology*. 2008;108(5):786-801.

Eipe N, Choudhrie A. Airway fires: gas-bugs providing the fuel [Letter]? *Anesth Analg*. 2005;101(5):1563-1564.

Talley HC. Anesthesia complications. In: Nagelhout JJ, Plaus KL, eds. *Nurse Anesthesia*. 4th ed. St Louis, MO: Saunders Elsevier; 2010:1302-1317.

Welliver MD, Welliver DC. Vocal cord polyp removal with laser. In: Elisha S, ed. *Case Studies in Nurse Anesthesia*. Sudbury, MA: Jones & Bartlett; 2011:41-50.

Chapter 4
Airway Obstruction

Treatment

Preoperative Management
- Complete a thorough preoperative airway assessment.
- Maintain spontaneous ventilation if the possibility of a difficult airway exists.
- Evaluate for causes of airway obstruction (see Table 4.1).
- Determine if the patient has a mediastinal mass causing airway obstruction.
- If superior vena cava syndrome exists, place IV in lower extremity.
- Prepare difficult airway adjuncts.

Intraoperative Management
- Increase FIO_2 to 100%.
- Suction airway and/or endotracheal tube.
- Identify and remove obstruction.
- Auscultate for clear, equal, and bilateral lung sounds.
- Reposition the head and neck using head-tilt, chin-lift method.
- Provide jaw-thrust maneuver.
- Insert nasopharyngeal or oropharyngeal airway device.
- Attempt 2-person ventilation.
- Consider supralaryngeal device (ie, LMA).
- Follow recommendations in the ASA difficult airway algorithm as indicated.
- Avoid muscle relaxation if tracheal or intrathoracic mass.

Treatment (continued)

- Consider cardiopulmonary bypass with a mediastinal mass that potentially impinges on airway structures.
- Consider rigid bronchoscopy for oxygenation and ventilation.
- Change patient position (semirecumbent, sitting, or lateral) for mediastinal mass–induced airway obstruction.

Postoperative Management

- Adjust F_{IO_2} to maintain saturation > 90%.
- Consider the use of noninvasive positive pressure ventilation device (CPAP or BiPAP).
- Monitor ABG results as needed.
- Obtain cervical and chest radiograph.
- Consider reintubation for patients in whom respiratory distress develops.
- Follow recommendations in the ASA difficult airway algorithm as indicated.
- Consider inhaled racemic epinephrine treatment and IV corticosteroids for upper airway edema.

Physiology and Pathophysiology

Airway obstruction can occur throughout the perioperative period and is caused by a variety of factors, as shown in Table 4.1. Obstruction in the upper and/or lower airway leads to impaired ventilation, decreased tissue oxygenation, and decreased removal of carbon dioxide. If hypoxia and/or hypercarbia ensue, a sympathetic nervous system response will predominate as a compensatory response to

Physiology and Pathophysiology (continued)

increase oxygen delivery to vital organs. Ultimately, if the cause of the airway obstruction is not identified and treated, hypoxia will eventually cause cerebral and myocardial tissue ischemia/infarction.

Table 4.1. Causes of Airway Obstruction

Upper airway	Lower airway
Tongue (most common)	ARDS
Anaphylaxis	Aspiration of foreign body
Aspiration of foreign body	Asthma
Burns	Bronchospasm
Hemoptysis	Burns (smoke and chemical inhalation)
Hemorrhage	COPD
Hypotension	Hemoptysis
Infection (laryngotracheo-bronchitis, epiglottitis, Ludwig angina, peritonsillar or retropharyngeal abscess)	Hemorrhage
Kink in ETT or circuit	Infection (pneumonia or tuberculosis)
Laryngeal or tracheal mass	Intrathoracic mass
Laryngospasm	Mediastinal mass
Mucous plug	Mucous plug
Obesity	Obesity
Obstructive sleep apnea	Pneumothorax
Surgical complications (eg, hematoma)	Pulmonary edema (CHF)
Tonsillar hypertrophy	Surgical complications (eg, hematoma)

Abbreviations: CHF, congestive heart failure; ARDS, acute respiratory distress syndrome; COPD, chronic obstructive pulmonary disease; ETT, endotracheal tube.

Table 4.1. Causes of Airway Obstruction (continued)

Upper airway	Lower airway
Trauma	Tension pneumothorax
Tumor	Trauma
Vocal cord polyp or papilloma	

Abbreviations: CHF, congestive heart failure; ARDS, acute respiratory distress syndrome; COPD, chronic obstructive pulmonary disease; ETT, endotracheal tube.

Signs and Symptoms

Respiratory
- Accessory muscle use during respiration
- Cyanosis
- Dyspnea
- Hemoptysis
- Hypercarbia
- Hypoxemia
- Subcutaneous emphysema
- Tachypnea

Upper Airway Obstruction
- Angioedema
- Barky cough
- Burned nose hairs
- High peak airway pressure
- Infection
- Radiographic evidence of obstruction
- Skin rash and/or pruritus (allergic reaction and/or anaphylaxis)
- Snoring
- Stridor
- Substernal retractions
- Tissue trauma
- Tracheal deviation
- Upper airway mass

Lower Airway Obstruction
- Abnormal breath sounds during auscultation (eg, wheezing, rales, or crackles)
- Absence of breath sounds
- High peak airway pressure
- Infection
- Radiographic evidence of obstruction
- Thoracic or substernal mass
- Tissue trauma

Signs and Symptoms (continued)

Cardiovascular
- Cardiac dysrhythmias
- Hypertension and tachycardia (early signs)
- Hypotension and bradycardia (late signs)

Neurologic
- Altered level of consciousness (agitation)

Differential Diagnosis

Respiratory
- ARDS
- Bronchospasm (see Chapter 8)
- ETT considerations
  - ETT malposition
  - Accidental extubation
  - ETT kinking
  - Mucous plug
  - Unidentified esophageal intubation
- Laryngeal edema
- Laryngospasm (see Chapter 25)
- Obstructive sleep apnea
- Oral or nasal airway malposition
- Pulmonary edema (eg, CHF)
- Pulmonary embolism (see Chapter 17)
- Retained pharyngeal and/or nasopharyngeal packing
- Secretions
- Sleep apnea
- Tracheomalacia

Cardiovascular
- Hypotension (see Chapter 22)

Neurologic
- Increased intracranial pressure
- Nerve damage or blockade
  - Phrenic nerve
  - Recurrent laryngeal nerve

Musculoskeletal
- Congenital craniofacial and airway abnormalities
- Facial, neck, or chest mass (eg, thyroid goiter)

Differential Diagnosis (continued)

Pharmacologic
- Pharmacologic considerations:
  - Alcohol intoxication
  - Excessive opioid, benzodiazepine, or propofol administration
  - Illicit depressant drug intoxication (eg, marijuana, heroin)

Other Considerations
- Anaphylaxis (see Chapter 5)
- Circuit disconnect
- Equipment malfunction
  - Capnography
  - Pulse oximetry
- Infection
  - Epiglottitis
  - Laryngotracheobronchitis
  - Pneumonia
  - Tuberculosis
- Trauma (airway, facial, or thoracic disruption)

Suggested Readings

Chipas A, Ellis WE. Airway management. In: Nagelhout JJ, Plaus KL, eds. *Nurse Anesthesia.* 4th ed. St Louis, MO: Saunders Elsevier; 2010: 441-464.

Mason RA, Fielder CP. The obstructed airway in head and neck surgery. *Anaesthesia.* 1999;54(7):625-628.

Welliver MD, Welliver DC. Vocal cord polyp removal with laser. In: Elisha S, ed. *Case Studies in Nurse Anesthesia.* Sudbury, MA: Jones & Bartlett; 2011:41-50.

Chapter 5
Anaphylaxis

Primary Interventions

- Discontinue suspected causative agent(s).
- Maintain patent airway and adequate ventilation.
- Call for help.
- Monitor for the presence of rapidly developing airway edema and obstruction.
- Administer 100% F_{IO_2}.
- Discontinue inhalation anesthetics.
- Confirm adequate IV access.
- Administer fluid bolus to treat hypotension.
- Give epinephrine IV (10-100 μg) for hypotension.
- Follow current ACLS or PALS guidelines as indicated.

Secondary Interventions

- Antihistamine: diphenhydramine IV (0.5-1 mg/kg)
- Vasopressor and inotropic medication infusion as needed
    - Epinephrine (4-8 μg/min)
    - Norepinephrine (4-8 μg/min)
    - Isoproterenol (0.5-1 μg/min)
- Bronchodilators: albuterol, terbutaline, and/or anticholinergic agents for persistent bronchospasm
- Corticosteroids: hydrocortisone IV (0.25-1 g) or equivalent
- Sodium bicarbonate IV (0.5-1 mEq/kg) for persistent hypotension or acidosis
- Vasopressin IV (40 U) for refractory shock

Treatment (continued)

- Consider invasive monitoring, as indicated.
- Monitor and manage acid-base status.
- Consider administering glucagon (1-2 mg) every 5 minutes for refractory anaphylaxis.

Physiology and Pathophysiology

Anaphylaxis is a type 1 hypersensitivity reaction caused by the degranulation of sensitized mast cells and basophils after exposure to an antigen. Mast cells are located in the perivascular spaces of the skin, lung, and intestine, and basophils are located in the blood. Upon initial exposure to an antigen, IgE is produced and binds to the surface of the effector cell. With subsequent exposure, the antigen binds to the IgE antibodies, releasing physiologically active mediators that include histamine, tryptase, chemotactic factors, and platelet-activating factor. Furthermore, metabolites such as prostaglandins, kinins, leukotrienes, and cytokines are synthesized and released. This results in a series of potentially life-threatening symptoms occurring most notably in the respiratory, cardiovascular, and integumentary systems. It is possible for an anaphylactic reaction to occur on first exposure to anesthetic medications because of cross-reactivity among many drugs and commercial household products.

In an *anaphylactoid reaction,* IgE is not produced. No previous sensitization is needed to trigger anaphylactoid reactions, and the results are clinically indistinguishable. The time of onset and the degree of clinical manifestations can vary greatly, making diagnosis complicated. In addition, many symptoms may be masked by general anesthesia and the use of surgical drapes, which conceal the cutaneous signs. Table 5.1 lists the agents that most commonly cause anaphylaxis.

Table 5.1. Agents Commonly Implicated in Anaphylactic Reactions

Agent	Incidence (%)
Neuromuscular blocking agents	58.2
Latex	16.7
Antibiotics	15.1
Colloids	4.0
Hypnotics	3.4
Opioids	1.3
Other agents	1.3

Signs and Symptoms

Respiratory
- Acute respiratory failure
- Bronchospasm
- Changes in voice quality
- Chest discomfort
- Coughing
- Cyanosis
- Decreased oxygen saturation
- Dyspnea
- Increased ETCO$_2$
- Increased PIP
- Laryngeal edema
- Sneezing
- Wheezing

Cardiovascular
- Cardiac arrest
- Chest discomfort
- Diaphoresis
- Dizziness
- Dysrhythmias
- Hypotension
- Malaise
- Tachycardia

Other Considerations
- Burning
- Flushing
- Itching
- Perioral edema
- Periorbital edema
- Tingling
- Urticaria (hives)

Differential Diagnosis

Respiratory
- Airway obstruction (see Chapter 4)
- Bronchospasm (see Chapter 8)
- Hypercarbia
- Hypoxia (see Chapter 24)
- Laryngospasm (see Chapter 25)
- Pneumothorax (see Chapter 31)
- Pulmonary edema
- Pulmonary embolism (see Chapter 17)
- Stridor (see Chapter 35)

Cardiovascular
- Cardiac dysrhythmias (see Chapter 9)
- Cardiac tamponade (see Chapter 10)
- Hereditary angioedema
- Hypotension (see Chapter 22)
- Myocardial ischemia or myocardial infarction (see Chapter 28)
- Shock (see Chapter 34)
- Vasovagal reaction
- Venous air embolism (see Chapter 17)
- Venous obstruction

Gastrointestinal
- Acute gastric aspiration (see Chapter 2)
- Esophageal or endobronchial intubation

Pharmacologic
- Direct histamine release (eg, morphine sulfate, atracurium)
- Discontinuation or overdose of vasodilator drug infusion
- Local anesthetic toxicity (see Chapter 26)

Other Considerations
- Electrolyte abnormalities (see Chapter 16)
- Mastocytosis

Suggested Readings

Levy JH. Immune function and allergic response. In: Barash PG, Cullen BF, Stoelting RK, Cahalan MK, Stock MC, eds. *Clinical Anesthesia*. 6th ed. Philadelphia, PA: Lippincott Williams & Wilkins; 2009:256-270.

Moss J. Allergic to anesthetics. *Anesthesiology*. 2003;99(3):521-523.

O'Donnell MP. The immune system and anesthesia. In: Nagelhout JJ, Plaus KL, eds. *Nurse Anesthesia*. 4th ed. St Louis, MO: Saunders Elsevier; 2010:985-1008.

Chapter 6
Anesthesia Machine Malfunction

Treatment

Primary Interventions
- Perform preanesthesia machine check.
- Identify and immediately repair malfunction.
- If necessary, obtain functional anesthesia machine for patient care.

Intraoperative Malfunction
- Call for help.
- Notify surgeon.
- If necessary, stop surgical procedure.
- Maintain adequate airway, breathing, and circulation.
- Systematically assess patient and anesthesia delivery system.
- If malfunction cannot be immediately determined, connect the patient to backup ventilation equipment for manual ventilation (eg, auxiliary oxygen cylinder and self-inflating manual ventilation device).
- For an anesthetized patient, ensure delivery of anesthesia via TIVA.
- If necessary, obtain backup anesthesia machine.

Postoperative Repair
- Contact company representative for servicing of anesthesia machine.

Physiology and Pathophysiology

The functions of an anesthesia machine are to assist the anesthesia provider with (1) oxygenation and ventilation of the patient, (2) carbon dioxide absorption, (3) inhaled anesthetic delivery, and (4) the safe removal of waste anesthetic gases from the scavenging system. Advanced technology has contributed to the rapid development of the modern anesthesia delivery system. Many newer anesthesia workstations are very complex (ie, with digital interfacing, internalized components, and computer software) and will require continual maintenance and system updates. Therefore, it is imperative that anesthesia providers be vigilant and maintain a detailed understanding of the anesthesia delivery system to provide safe patient care. Figure 6.1 illustrates the basic functional structure of the anesthesia delivery system, which includes the following:

1. Gas delivery system: gas supply source, pressure-regulating valves, fail-safe valves, oxygen low-pressure alarm, gas mixing components, and inhalation anesthetic vaporizers
2. Patient breathing system: anesthesia breathing circuit, carbon dioxide absorber, inspiratory and expiratory valves, and mechanical ventilator
3. Waste inhalation anesthetic scavenging system
4. Integrated patient physiological monitoring systems

Malfunction of the anesthesia delivery system can occur at any level of this functional structure (Table 6.1). The low-pressure circuit is the "vulnerable area" of an anesthesia machine because (1) it is most subject to breakage and leaks, (2) it is located downstream from all safety features except the oxygen analyzer, and (3) inappropriate low-pressure circuit testing will not detect malfunctions in this area. Manual and automated checklists function to assess the integrity of the anesthesia delivery system. Preanesthesia checkout procedures must be performed before every anesthetic delivered. Table 6.2 provides recommendations for preanesthesia checkout procedures.

Figure 6.1. Basic Functional Structure of the Anesthesia Machine

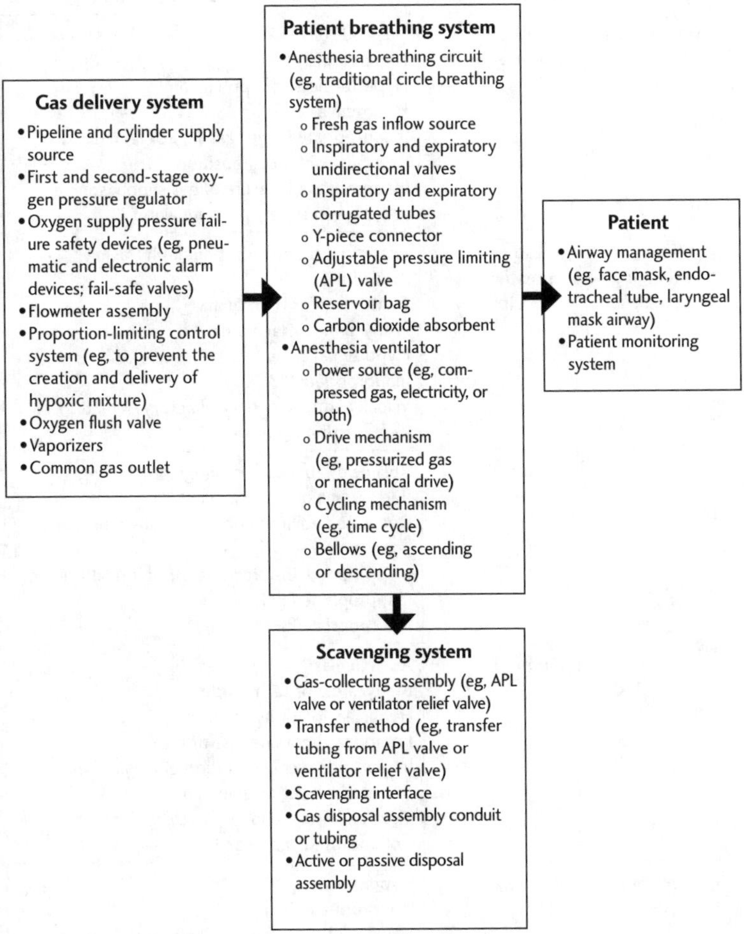

Patient breathing system
- Anesthesia breathing circuit (eg, traditional circle breathing system)
  - o Fresh gas inflow source
  - o Inspiratory and expiratory unidirectional valves
  - o Inspiratory and expiratory corrugated tubes
  - o Y-piece connector
  - o Adjustable pressure limiting (APL) valve
  - o Reservoir bag
  - o Carbon dioxide absorbent
- Anesthesia ventilator
  - o Power source (eg, compressed gas, electricity, or both)
  - o Drive mechanism (eg, pressurized gas or mechanical drive)
  - o Cycling mechanism (eg, time cycle)
  - o Bellows (eg, ascending or descending)

Gas delivery system
- Pipeline and cylinder supply source
- First and second-stage oxygen pressure regulator
- Oxygen supply pressure failure safety devices (eg, pneumatic and electronic alarm devices; fail-safe valves)
- Flowmeter assembly
- Proportion-limiting control system (eg, to prevent the creation and delivery of hypoxic mixture)
- Oxygen flush valve
- Vaporizers
- Common gas outlet

Patient
- Airway management (eg, face mask, endotracheal tube, laryngeal mask airway)
- Patient monitoring system

Scavenging system
- Gas-collecting assembly (eg, APL valve or ventilator relief valve)
- Transfer method (eg, transfer tubing from APL valve or ventilator relief valve)
- Scavenging interface
- Gas disposal assembly conduit or tubing
- Active or passive disposal assembly

Table 6.1. Malfunctions Associated With the Anesthesia Machine

Delivery system	Malfunction	Signs and symptoms
Gas delivery system	Gas supply source	F_{IO_2} < 30% Hypercarbia Hypertension or hypotension Hypoxemia Inappropriate carrier gas (eg, oxygen, air, or nitrous oxide) composition Inappropriate pressure of gas supply source Low oxygen supply pressure alarm
Patient breathing system	Anesthesia breathing circuit	Absent or abnormal capnograph tracing Arrhythmias Barotrauma or volutrauma Bradycardia or tachycardia Hypoxemia Inappropriate PIP Visual, auditory, and/or olfactory detection of anesthetic gas leak
	Unidirectional valves	Absent or abnormal capnography tracing Barotrauma or volutrauma Decreased ability to provide positive pressure ventilation Inappropriate inspired and expired tidal volume Inappropriate PEEP Inappropriate PIP
	Vaporizer	Arrhythmias Bradycardia or tachycardia Hypertension or hypotension Intraoperative awareness or recall Inappropriate concentration of inspired or expired inhalation anesthetic Visual, auditory, and/or olfactory detection of anesthetic gas leak
Scavenging system	Scavenging system	Hypoxemia Inappropriate PEEP Visual, auditory, and/or olfactory detection of anesthetic gas leak

Abbreviations: F_{IO_2}, fraction of inspired oxygen; PIP, peak inspiratory pressure; PEEP, positive end-expiratory pressure.

Table 6.2. Recommendations for Preanesthesia Checkout Procedures

Verify that emergency ventilation equipment (eg, oxygen cylinder and self-inflating manual ventilation device) is available and functioning.

Verify that patient suction is adequate to clear secretions and blood from the airway.

Turn on master switch to anesthesia delivery system and confirm that electrical power is available.

Check, calibrate, and set alarm limits for all physiological monitors.

Check oxygen cylinder supply and verify that pressure is adequate on the emergency oxygen cylinder mounted on the anesthesia machine.

Check central pipeline supplies and verify that the piped gas pressures are > 50 PSI.

Verify that vaporizers are adequately filled and the filler ports are tightly closed.

Test flowmeters and verify the appropriate movement of the bobbins or floats.

Perform leak check of low-pressure system and confirm that there are no leaks in the gas supply between the flowmeters and the common gas outlet.

Adjust and check the scavenging system function.

Calibrate the oxygen monitor and check the low oxygen alarm.

Verify that the carbon dioxide absorbent is not exhausted.

Perform a leak check of the patient breathing system.

Test the patient ventilation system and unidirectional valves to verify that gas flows properly through the breathing circuit during inhalation and exhalation.

Document completion of checkout procedures.

Confirm ventilator settings and evaluate readiness to deliver anesthesia care.

Check final status of anesthesia delivery system.

Perform anesthesia time out.

Abbreviation: PSI, pounds per square inch.
Adapted from FDA guidelines for an anesthesia machine check procedure.

Signs and Symptoms

Respiratory
- Absent, increased, or other abnormality of exhaled carbon dioxide concentration on the capnography tracing
- Barotrauma or volutrauma
- Decreased ability to provide positive pressure ventilation
- Desaturation
- $F_{IO_2} < 30\%$
- Hypercarbia
- Hypoxia
- Inappropriate inspired and expired tidal volume
- Inappropriate PEEP
- Inappropriate PIP

Cardiovascular
- Dysrhythmias
- Hypertension or hypotension
- Tachycardia or bradycardia

Pharmacologic
- Inappropriate carrier gas (eg, oxygen, air, or nitrous oxide) composition
- Inappropriate concentration of inspired or expired inhalation anesthetic

Other Considerations
- Inappropriate pressure of gas supply source
- Intraoperative patient awareness or recall
- Low oxygen supply pressure alarm
- Malfunction during preanesthesia checkout procedure
- Visual, auditory, and/or olfactory detection of anesthetic gas leak
- See Table 6.1 for other specific malfunctions.

Differential Diagnosis

Respiratory
- Airway and/or operating room fire (see Chapter 3)
- Bronchospasm (see Chapter 8)
- Endobronchial intubation
- Hypoxia, actual or related to mechanical malfunction or inaccuracy (see Chapter 24)
- Pneumothorax (see Chapter 31)

Cardiovascular
- Embolic event (see Chapter 17)
- Hypercarbia (see Chapter 19)
- Hypertension (see Chapter 20)
- Hypotension (see Chapter 22)

Other Considerations
- Carbon dioxide absorber exhaustion

Suggested Readings

Caplan RA, Vistica MF, Posner KL, Cheney FW. Adverse anesthetic outcomes arising from gas delivery equipment: a closed claims analysis. *Anesthesiology*. 1997;87(4):741-748.

Fasting S, Gisvold SE. Equipment problems during anaesthesia: are they a quality problem? *Br J Anaesth*. 2002;89(6):825-831.

Waldrop WB, Murray DJ, Boulet JR, Kras JF. Management of anesthesia equipment failure: a simulation-based resident skill assessment. *Anesth Analg*. 2009;109(2):426-433.

Chapter 7
Autonomic Hyperreflexia

Treatment

- Inform surgeon.
- Stop surgery when appropriate.
- Eliminate noxious stimulus.
- Increase anesthetic depth.
- Administer 1 or more IV vasodilator(s) and titrate to desired effect:
    - Nitroprusside
    - Nitroglycerin
    - Hydralazine
    - Trimethaphan
    - Phentolamine
- Insert arterial line.
- Manage neurologic, cardiac, and pulmonary manifestations associated with hypertension.
- Administer neuraxial anesthesia (eg, epidural) if autonomic hyperreflexia is caused by uterine contractions.
- Obtain central venous access and CVP monitoring.

Physiology and Pathophysiology

Autonomic hyperreflexia, or dysreflexia, describes the sudden sympathetic nervous system response that occurs after a chronic spinal

Physiology and Pathophysiology (continued)

cord transection. Initiation of this condition has been observed in up to 85% of patients with spinal cord injury above the level of T6. The classic presentation associated with autonomic hyperreflexia includes the following:

- Systemic hypertension
- Bradycardia
- Cutaneous vasodilation above the level of the spinal cord transection

Noxious stimulation below the level of a spinal cord injury activates sensory impulses, which causes (1) a sympathetic nervous system response, (2) vasoconstriction of the splanchnic circulation, and (3) an increase in systemic blood pressure. In neurologically intact patients, this sympathetic response is modulated by higher neurologic centers. In patients with a complete spinal cord transection, neurologic modulation is isolated from the sympathetic response and vasoconstriction persists below the level of the injury. In addition, the increase in systemic blood pressure activates central and peripheral baroreceptors causing bradycardia and cutaneous vasodilation above the level of the spinal cord transection.

Signs and Symptoms

Respiratory
- Dyspnea
- Hypoxemia
- Pulmonary edema
- Rales
- Rhonchi

Cardiovascular
- Cardiac dysrhythmias
- CHF
- Classic presentation:

o Bradycardia
o Cutaneous vasodilation above the level of the spinal cord transection (piloerection, sweating, nasal congestion, or cutaneous flushing)
o Hypertension
- Myocardial infarction or ischemia

Signs and Symptoms (continued)

Neurologic
- Altered level of consciousness
- Blurred vision
- Cerebral herniation
- Cerebral vascular accident
- Cushing triad (eg, hypertension, bradycardia, irregular respiration)
- Headache
- Intracranial hemorrhage
- Seizures

Differential Diagnosis

Respiratory
- Pulmonary edema

Cardiovascular
- Hypertension (see Chapter 20)

Neurologic
- Increased intracranial pressure
  - o Intracranial neoplasm
  - o Neurovascular pathology
  - o Traumatic brain injury
- Neuroleptic malignant syndrome
- Noxious stimulus below level of spinal cord transection
  - o Cutaneous and/or visceral stimulation (eg, surgery, temperature extremes)
  - o Distention of a hollow organ (bladder, uterus, or rectum)
  - o Intense smooth muscle contraction (eg, uterine contractions)
- Pain

Endocrine
- Carcinoid syndrome
- Pheochromocytoma
- Thyrotoxicosis

Pharmacologic
- Acute drug intoxication (eg, stimulants, cocaine, and/or amphetamines)
- Cholinergic crisis

Differential Diagnosis (continued)

- Excessive adrenergic receptor agonist administration and/or medication error (phenylephrine or epinephrine)

- Malignant hyperthermia
- Preeclampsia or eclampsia in parturient with spinal cord transection

Other Considerations
- Inadequate depth of anesthesia

Suggested Readings

Barton CR, Radesic BP. Trauma anesthesia. In: Nagelhout JJ, Plaus KL, eds. *Nurse Anesthesia.* 4th ed. St Louis, MO: Saunders Elsevier; 2010:875-891.

Hebl JR, Horlocker TT, Schroeder DR. Neuraxial anesthesia and analgesia in patients with preexisting central nervous system disorders. *Anesth Analg.* 2006;103(1):223-228.

Heiner JS. Penetrating traumatic injuries. In: Elisha S, ed. *Case Studies in Nurse Anesthesia.* Sudbury, MA: Jones & Bartlett; 2011:167-179.

Chapter 8
Bronchospasm

- Maintain a secure and patent airway.
- Provide F_{IO_2} at 100%.
- Ventilate manually.
- Diagnose and treat underlying mechanical or pathological cause.

Mild to Moderate Bronchospasm (adequate ventilation and acceptable oxygen saturation)
- Increase inhalational anesthetic concentration.
- Increase anesthetic depth (eg, propofol, narcotics).
- Administer albuterol via nebulizer or metered-dose inhaler.

Severe Bronchospasm (difficulty or inability to ventilate, unacceptable oxygen saturation, and persistent signs and symptoms)
- Call for help.
- Stop surgery.
- Treatment as indicated above.
- Administer bronchodilators:
  1. Epinephrine IV bolus (1-10 μg/kg) titrated to effect
  2. Epinephrine IV infusion (1-4 μg/min)
  3. Terbutaline SQ (0.5 mg)
  4. Magnesium sulfate IV infusion (2 g over 10 minutes)
  5. Aminophylline IV (loading dose, 6 mg/kg; infusion, 0.5-0.7 mg/kg/h)
- Administer corticosteroids (hydrocortisone IV [0.25-1 g] or equivalent).

Treatment (continued)

- Ventilate using high-pressure ICU ventilator.
- Assess adequacy of treatment and acid-base status as needed (eg, ABG measurement).

Physiology and Pathophysiology

Bronchospasm is an acute and reversible narrowing of the broncho-pulmonary segments. Wheezing, a common finding during broncho-spasm, is a result of turbulent airflow through these narrowed segments causing increased airway resistance. Increased airway reactivity in specific populations (eg, smokers, and persons with COPD) may predispose the patients to bronchospastic episodes. During anesthesia, bronchospasm is most often caused by physiological stimulation (eg, airway manipulation, endotracheal tube stimulation, surgical stimulation, light anesthesia). Treatment includes (1) maintaining adequate ventilation and oxygenation, (2) increasing anesthetic depth, (3) administering bronchodilators and (4) identifying and treating the underlying mechanical or pathological cause. It also can occur because of histamine release caused by medication (eg, atracurium, morphine sulfate).

"Shark fin" morphology of the end-tidal carbon dioxide waveform (eg, decreased or slanted expiratory limb) is characteristic of mild to moderate bronchospasm due to air trapping from bronchoconstriction and is shown in Figure 8.1. During severe episodes of bronchospasm, inadequate ventilation or the absence of ventilation may manifest as an absent $ETCO_2$ waveform. As with any disease process, it is imperative to exclude other potential causes (eg, circuit disconnection or obstructed airway) before initiating treatment.

Figure 8.1. Sloped Expiratory Limb on the ETCO$_2$ Capnography Waveform Consistent with Bronchospasm

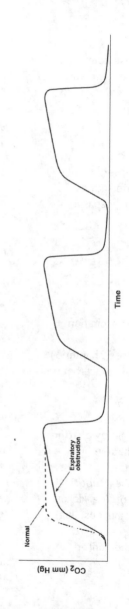

Signs and Symptoms

Respiratory
- Decreased bag compliance during manual ventilation
- Decreased breath sounds
- Desaturation
- Hypercarbia
- Hypoxia
- Increased PIP
- Minimal or absent ETCO$_2$ and/or breath sounds (severe bronchospasm)
- Sloped expiratory limb on ETCO$_2$ waveform (mild to moderate bronchospasm)
- Wheezing

Cardiovascular
- Cardiac arrest
- Dysrhythmias
- Hypertension
- Tachycardia

Differential Diagnosis

Respiratory
- Acute gastric aspiration (see Chapter 2)
- Airway fire (see Chapter 3)
- Asthma, acute exacerbation
- COPD
- Laryngospasm (see Chapter 25)
- Mechanical airway obstruction (see Chapter 4)
    1. Secretions
    2. Endotracheal tube obstruction (eg, kinking, biting, or mucous plug)
    3. Breathing circuit restricted or kinked
- Pneumothorax (see Chapter 31)
- Pressure from the ETT on the carina
- Pulmonary edema
- Pulmonary embolism (see Chapter 17)
- Upper respiratory tract infection

Pharmacologic
- Airway-irritating inhalation agent (eg, desflurane)
- Anticholinesterase agents
- Antiprostaglandin agents (eg, ketorolac)
- β-Blocking medications

Differential Diagnosis (continued)

- Medications associated with histamine release (eg, atracurium, morphine)
- Propofol preparations that contain metabisulfite

Other Considerations
- Anaphylaxis (see Chapter 5)
- Carcinoid syndrome
- Endobronchial intubation
- Endotracheal tube touching the carina
- Light anesthesia and/or surgical stimulation

Suggested Readings

Kant A, McKinlay J. Severe bronchospasm or anaphylaxis? *Anaesthesia.* 2010;65(1):90-91.

Talley HC. Anesthesia complications. In: Nagelhout JJ, Plaus KL, eds. *Nurse Anesthesia.* 4th ed. St Louis, MO: Saunders Elsevier; 2010:1302-1317.

Yao FSF. Asthma and chronic obstructive pulmonary disease. In: Yao FSF, Malhotra V, Fontes ML, eds. *Yao & Artusio's Anesthesiology: Problem-Oriented Patient Management.* 6th ed. Philadelphia, PA: Lippincott Williams & Wilkins; 2008:1-28.

Chapter 9
Cardiac Dysrhythmias

Treatment

- Identify presence of cardiac dysrhythmia in 2 leads (eg, II and V5).
- Assess for hemodynamic instability:
  - Altered level of consciousness
  - Hypotension
  - Loss of central and/or peripheral pulses
  - Myocardial infarction or ischemia
  - Pulmonary edema
  - CHF
  - Hypoxemia
- Follow current American Heart Association ACLS or PALS guidelines.
- Provide 100% oxygen.
- Treat underlying pathological cause.
- Provide supportive measures as needed:
  - Airway management and intubation
  - Invasive monitoring (eg, arterial line, central line)
  - Vasopressor medication(s)
  - Inotropic medication(s)
  - Antidysrhythmic medication(s)
- Obtain 12-lead ECG as needed.
- Consult with a cardiologist as needed.
- See Table 9.1 for symptoms, differential diagnosis, and treatment of specific cardiac dysrhythmias.
- Perform cardiac resuscitation per ACLS or PALS protocol as necessary.

Physiology and Pathophysiology

During the course of a normal cardiac cycle, the conduction pathways and structural components of the heart work in coordination. This synchrony is vital to venous blood oxygenation and, ultimately, oxygen delivery to peripheral and central tissues. Cardiac dysrhythmias can be precipitated by physiological stress and can occur when myocardial oxygen demand exceeds supply. This imbalance can cause conduction and/or structural aberrancies that are associated with the cardiac cycle. Medical management includes antidysrhythmic medication, antithrombotic medication, pacemaker insertion, and automatic implantable cardioverter-defibrillator efficacy. The severity of a particular cardiac dysrhythmia is dependent on the following:

- Etiology
- Onset and duration (acute or chronic presentation)
- Effect on venous blood oxygenation and oxygen delivery
- Adequacy of preoperative medical management

See Table 9.1 for specific information for the following cardiac dysrhythmias:

1. Sinus bradycardia and AV heart block
2. Sinus tachycardia
3. Atrial tachyarrhythmias (eg, atrial fibrillation, atrial flutter, supraventricular tachycardia)
4. Ventricular tachyarrhythmias (eg, ventricular tachycardia, ventricular fibrillation, torsades de pointes)
5. Pulseless electrical activity and asystole

The differential diagnosis and treatment of cardiac dysrhythmias should be based on treating the underlying pathological state and instituting ACLS or PALS guidelines.

Table 9.1. Cardiac Dysrhythmias: Symptoms, Differential Diagnosis, and Treatment

Cardiac dysrhythmia	Signs and symptoms	Differential diagnosis	Treatment
Bradycardia	Sinus bradycardia heart rate < 60/min First-, second-, and third-degree AV nodal block	Conduction disease Structural disease Perioperative stress 8 Hs and 8 Ts (see page 49)	ACLS or PALS Epinephrine Atropine Transcutaneous pacing Dopamine
Tachycardia	Sinus tachycardia heart rate > 100/min	Conduction disease Structural disease Perioperative stress 8 Hs and 8 Ts	Increase depth of anesthesia Provide analgesia Assess for hypovolemia Assess for hypermetabolic pathological state
Atrial tachydys-rhythmias	Atrial fibrillation and flutter SVT	Conduction disease Structural disease Perioperative stress 8 Hs and 8 Ts	ACLS or PALS Atrial fibrillation and flutter Synchronized cardioversion Rate control with diltiazem, β-blockers, or digoxin SVT Vagal maneuvers (carotid massage) Rate control with adenos-ine, diltiazem, or β-blockers
Ventricular tachydys-rhythmias	VT and VF Torsades de pointes	Conduction disease Structural disease Perioperative stress 8 Hs and 8 Ts	ACLS or PALS VT Biphasic defibrillation Epinephrine Vasopressin Amiodarone Lidocaine Torsades de pointes Magnesium sulfate
PEA and asystole	PEA Asystole	Conduction disease Structural disease Perioperative stress 8 Hs and 8 Ts	ACLS or PALS Epinephrine Vasopressin Atropine

Abbreviations: AV, atrial ventricular; ACLS, advanced cardiac life support; PALS, pediatric advanced life support; SVT, supraventricular tachycardia; PEA, pulseless electrical activity; VT, ventricular tachycardia; VF, ventricular fibrillation.

Signs and Symptoms

Respiratory
- Dyspnea
- Hypoxemia
- Pulmonary edema

Cardiovascular
- Abnormal ECG identified in 2 leads (eg, II and V5)
- Cardiac dysrhythmias
- Chest pain
- CHF
- Hypotension
- Left ventricular dysfunction
- Loss of peripheral and/or central pulses
- Myocardial ischemia or infarction

Neurologic
- Altered level of consciousness and/or loss of consciousness
- Ischemic stroke

Gastrointestinal
- Nausea and/or vomiting

Other Considerations
- See Table 9.1 for symptoms, differential diagnosis, and treatment of specific cardiac dysrhythmias

Differential Diagnosis

Cardiovascular
- Conduction cardiac disease
  1. First-, second-, third-degree AV nodal block
  2. Fascicular block (eg, bundle branch block)
  3. Q-T interval prolongation
  4. Sinus node dysfunction (eg, sick sinus syndrome)
  5. WPW syndrome

- Structural cardiac disease
  1. Cardiomyopathy (eg, dilated cardiomyopathy)
  2. COPD
  3. Congenital cardiac disease
  4. CAD
  5. Inflammatory disease (eg, pericarditis)
  6. Postcardiac surgical intervention
  7. Valvular cardiac disease

Differential Diagnosis (continued)

Other Considerations
- Perioperative physiologic stress
  1. Induction and emergence of anesthesia
  2. Neuraxial anesthesia (eg, sympathectomy or high spinal anesthesia)
  3. Laryngoscopy and tracheal intubation
  4. Inadequate depth of anesthesia and analgesia
  5. Surgical stimulation and pain
  6. Medication overdose or error

"8 Hs"
  1. Hydrogen ion excess (eg, hypercarbia and acidosis)
  2. Hyperelectrolyte or hypo-electrolyte abnormalities (eg, sodium, potassium, calcium, and magnesium)
  3. Hypervagal parasympathetic predominance
  4. Hyperthermia (eg, malignant hyperthermia, see Chapter 27)
  5. Hypoglycemia
  6. Hypothermia (see Chapter 23)
  7. Hypovolemia
  8. Hypoxia (see Chapter 24)

"8 Ts"
  1. Tablets (eg, digitalis, droperidol, narcotics, β-blockers, calcium channel blockers)
  2. Tamponade, cardiac (see Chapter 10)
  3. Tension (pneumothorax, see Chapter 31)
  4. Thrombosis (eg, pulmonary embolus, see Chapter 17; myocardial infarction, see Chapter 28)
  5. Thyroid (eg, myxedema coma or thyrotoxicosis)
  6. Toxicity (eg, anaphylaxis, see Chapter 5; local anesthetic toxicity, see Chapter 26)
  7. Trauma (eg, shock states, see Chapter 34)
  8. Treatment, cancer (eg, anthracycline antibiotics such as doxorubicin)
- See Table 9.1 for signs and symptoms, differential diagnosis, and treatment of specific cardiac dysrhythmias.

Suggested Readings

Kossick MA. Antiarrhythmics. In: Ouellette RG, Joyce JA, eds. *Pharmacology for Nurse Anesthesiology.* Sudbury, MA: Jones & Bartlett; 2011:385-401.

Talley HC. Anesthesia complications. In: Nagelhout JJ, Plaus KL, eds. *Nurse Anesthesia.* 4th ed. St Louis, MO: Saunders Elsevier; 2010:1302-1317.

Thompson A, Balser JR. Perioperative cardiac arrhythmias. *Br J Anaesth.* 2004;93(1):86-94.

Chapter 10
Cardiac Tamponade

Treatment

- Maintain normal or slightly elevated heart rate.
- Hemodynamics:
  - Maintain preload (crystalloid, colloid, or blood).
  - Avoid fluid overload.
  - Avoid increases in afterload.
- Increase FIO_2 to keep SpO_2 > 90%.
- Intubate if respiratory distress occurs.
- Insert an arterial line.
- Consider CVP and intracardiac pressure monitoring.
- Place 2 large-bore peripheral IV lines.
- Avoid increases in intrathoracic pressure (PEEP and/or high PIP).
- Consider low tidal volumes and higher respiratory rates for ventilation.
- Assess and treat primary cause.
- Consider the presence of other injuries if cardiac tamponade is associated with trauma.
- Perform cardiac resuscitation per American Heart Association ACLS or PALS protocol as necessary.
- Perform diagnostic studies:
  - ECG
  - Echocardiogram
  - Chest radiograph

Treatment (continued)

- Interventions for cardiac tamponade:
  - Percutaneous pericardiocentesis
  - Pericardiotomy
  - Anterolateral thoracotomy

Physiology and Pathophysiology

Cardiac tamponade, also known as cardiac compressive shock, is the result of pressure on the heart that inhibits cardiac filling and contraction. This pathology is most commonly caused by pericardial effusion, which is an accumulation of fluid in the pericardial sac surrounding the heart. Pericardial effusions can result from an imbalance of fluid production and reabsorption or from structural abnormalities that allow excessive fluid to accumulate within the pericardial sac. The increase in pericardial pressure decreases the ability of the heart to relax and fill with blood, causing diastolic dysfunction. The result is an increase in CVP and a decrease in preload and cardiac output. Surgical procedures that are associated with an increased risk of cardiac tamponade include cardiac catheterization, cardiac revascularization, and pacemaker insertion.

The rate of fluid accumulation in the pericardial space determines the speed and severity of cardiac dysfunction. Normal pericardial fluid consists of 25 to 50 mL, and a rapid accumulation of only 100 to 200 mL can cause severe signs and symptoms associated with cardiac tamponade. However, with gradual accumulation of pericardial fluid, the pericardial fibers stretch and compensate for the increased volume. However, when a critical volume is reached, cardiac tamponade will occur.

Physiology and Pathophysiology (continued)

Cardiac tamponade may also occur as a result of a traumatic injury (eg, blunt force or penetrating trauma to the thorax, acceleration-deceleration injuries). Bleeding within the pericardial sac can originate from a laceration of coronary arteries or from perforation of the heart. Immediate intervention is necessary to avoid cardiovascular collapse.

Signs and Symptoms

Respiratory
- Cyanosis
- Hypercarbia
- Hypoxia
- Orthopnea
- Tachypnea

Cardiovascular
- Beck triad
  1. Hypotension
  2. Jugular venous distention
  3. Muffled heart sounds
- Cardiac arrest
- Cardiac dysrhythmias
- Chest pain or pressure
- Chest radiograph showing an enlarged cardiac shadow that appears globular
- Diastolic pressure equalization in all 4 cardiac chambers
- ECG changes (eg, evidence of ischemia)
- Echocardiography revealing fluid accumulation around the heart and diastolic collapse of the right atrium and right ventricle
- Increased CVP (early sign)
- Narrowed pulse pressure
- Pulseless electrical activity
- Pulsus paradoxus (decrease in systolic pressure of > 10 mm Hg during inspiration)
- Tachycardia

Neurologic
- Altered consciousness or loss of consciousness

Renal
- Oliguria

Differential Diagnosis

Respiratory
- Pulmonary edema
- Tension pneumothorax (see Chapter 31)

Cardiovascular
- Acute myocardial ischemia or infarction (see Chapter 28)
- Aortic dissection
- CHF
- Hemorrhage
- Hypovolemia
- Increased intrathoracic pressure (eg, PEEP)
- Superior vena cava syndrome

Musculoskeletal
- Connective tissue disorders
- Mediastinal mass

Pharmacologic
- Anaphylaxis (see Chapter 5)

Other Considerations
- All shock states (see Chapter 34)
- Bacterial infections (eg, tuberculosis)
- Trauma to the chest, or severe acceleration-deceleration injuries

Suggested Readings

Brouillette CV. Anesthesia for cardiac surgery. In: Nagelhout JJ, Plaus KL, eds. *Nurse Anesthesia.* 4th ed. St Louis, MO: Saunders Elsevier; 2010:504-527.

Soler -Soler J, Sagristà-Sauleda J, Permanyer-Miralda G. Management of pericardial effusion. *Heart.* 2001;86(2):235-240.

Spodick DH. Acute cardiac tamponade. *N Engl J Med.* 2003;349(7): 684-690.

Chapter 11
Complex Regional Pain Syndrome

Treatment

General Principles
- The goal is to achieve remission of syndrome.
- Severity of syndrome dictates treatment regimen.
- Focus is on restoration in physical functioning of the extremity.
- A multidisciplinary approach including pain management, physical and/or occupational therapy, and psychological and/or psychiatric treatment is necessary.
- Anesthetic recommendations:
  - Consider regional block on the affected limb before surgical stimulation.
  - Consider avoiding invasive and/or noninvasive blood pressure monitoring on the affected limb.

Specific Pain Management Modalities
- Pharmacologic:
  - Nonsteroidal anti-inflammatory drugs: naproxen and ibuprofen
  - Opioids: tramadol, morphine, and oxycodone
  - Tricyclic antidepressants: amitriptyline, desipramine, and maprotiline
  - Calcium and/or sodium channel anticonvulsants: gabapentin, pregabalin and/or carbamazepine, and lidocaine
  - Corticosteroids
- Invasive procedures:
  - Sympathetic nerve blocks to relieve symptoms and/or to identify if pain is sympathetic in nature
  - Spinal cord and/or peripheral nerve stimulation

Treatment (continued)

- Psychological and/or psychiatric:
  - Develop coping strategies.
  - Identify underlying psychological disorders.
- Physical and/or occupational therapy:
  - Isometric exercises
  - Gentle range of motion

Physiology and Pathophysiology

CRPS is a chronic neuropathic pain syndrome affecting the distal extremities. Its pathophysiological mechanisms, although uncertain, are multifactorial, with both peripheral and CNS involvement. Among these are (1) inflammation, (2) peripheral and central sensitization, (3) alterations in somatosensory processing, and (4) altered sympathetic and catecholaminergic function. CRPS tends to have an unpredictable clinical course, and a distinct plan for treatment must be individualized.

CRPS consists of 2 subtypes: type 1 (reflex sympathetic dystrophy) and type 2 (causalgia). CRPS type 1 develops after acute tissue trauma to an extremity without any apparent nerve injuries. CRPS type 2 develops after a known injury that has "caused" peripheral nerve damage. Clinical features include different symptoms that are associated with pain and sensory abnormalities, edema of the skin and subcutaneous tissues, vasomotor instability, autonomic abnormalities, and impaired motor function.

Signs and Symptoms

- Allodynia (pain caused by a normally nonpainful stimulus)
- Continuous pain that is disproportionate to the inciting event
- Decreased range of motion
- Discoloration and/or changes to the texture of hair, skin, or nails
- Dystonia
- Edema
- Hyperalgesia (an increased response to a stimulus that is normally painful)
- Hyperesthesia (increased perception of a nonnoxious stimulus)
- Myoclonus
- Pain described as burning, squeezing, throbbing, aching, shooting, and/or spreading beyond the area of initial injury, possibly involving the entire limb and rarely involving the contralateral limb
- Psychological symptoms (eg, depression, anxiety, or posttraumatic stress disorder)
- Skin abnormalities of affected extremity
- Sweating abnormalities
- Temperature abnormalities of affected extremity
- Tremor
- Weakness

Differential Diagnosis

Cardiovascular
- Cellulitis
- Deep vein thrombosis
- Lymphedema
- Peripheral vascular disease
- Posttraumatic vasoconstriction
- Thrombophlebitis
- Vascular insufficiency

Other Considerations
- Carpal tunnel syndrome
- Compartment syndrome
- Diabetic neuropathy
- Entrapment neuropathy
- Fibromyalgia
- Lateral epicondylitis (eg, tennis elbow)
- Peripheral neuropathy

Differential Diagnosis (continued)

Other Considerations
- Repetitive strain injury
- Shoulder-hand syndrome
- Thoracic outlet syndrome
- Undetected fracture

Suggested Readings

Albazaz R, Wong YT, Homer-Vanniasinkam S. Complex regional pain syndrome: a review. *Ann Vasc Surg.* 2008;22(2):297-306.

Binder A, Baron R. Complex regional pain syndrome, including applications of neural blockade. In: Cousins MJ, Carr DB, Horlocker TT, Bridenbaugh PO, eds. *Cousins & Bridenbaugh's Neural Blockade in Clinical Anesthesia and Pain Medicine.* 4th ed. Philadelphia, PA: Lippincott Williams & Wilkins; 2009:1154-1168.

Bruehl S. An update on the pathophysiology of complex regional pain syndrome. *Anesthesiology.* 2010;113(3):713-725.

Stanton-Hicks M. Complex regional pain syndrome. In: Warfield CA, Bajwa ZH, eds. *Principles & Practice of Pain Medicine.* 2nd ed. New York, NY: McGraw-Hill; 2004:405-416.

Chapter 12
Delayed Emergence

Treatment

- Maintain patent airway.
- Ensure adequate ventilation.
- Identify and treat cause.
- Use pharmacologic treatment as indicated:
  - Discontinue anesthetic mediation administration.
  - Nondepolarizing muscle relaxant reversal: anticholinesterase agent (eg, neostigmine) and anticholinergic
  - Narcotic reversal: naloxone IV (40 μg every 2 minutes up to 200 μg)
  - Benzodiazepine reversal: flumazenil IV (0.2 mg every minute up to 1 mg)
  - Hypoglycemia: 50% dextrose IV (25 g/50 mL)
  - Hyperglycemia: regular insulin by sliding scale
- Institute forced-air warming for hypothermia.
- Monitor ABG, electrolyte, and glucose values, and treat abnormalities appropriately.
- Consider serum or urine drug screen.
- Consider pseudocholinesterase deficiency if succinylcholine was administered.
- If increased intracranial pressure is suspected:
  - Request neurosurgical consult.
  - Treat increased intracranial pressure:
    - Correction of hypoxia and hypercarbia
    - Mild hyperventilation
    - Loop diuretic (eg, furosemide IV, 10-100 mg) or osmotic diuretic (eg, mannitol IV, 0.25-1 g/kg)

Treatment (continued)

- — Promotion of venous drainage with neutral head and/or neck position and head of bed elevated 45°
- — Surgical decompression (removal of space-occupying lesion, ventriculostomy drain, or lumbar intrathecal drain)
- — Corticosteroids (dexamethasone IV, 10-20 mg)
- — Intravenous fluid restriction
- Consider CT and MRI studies.
- Continue intensive care monitoring with periodic neurologic assessment.

Physiology and Pathophysiology

Delayed emergence occurs after anesthetic administration has been discontinued and the patient remains unconscious. Delayed emergence can be attributed to the following:

1. Prolonged pharmacological actions of anesthetic agents
2. Metabolic abnormalities
3. Inadequate cerebral perfusion
4. Neurologic injury

Delayed emergence is frequently caused by the residual cerebral depressant effects of anesthetic medications. This may be the result of excessive drug administration, synergistic effects between CNS depressants, or alterations in drug pharmacokinetic and/or pharmacodynamic profiles based on genetic or environmental factors. Pharmacokinetic drug action can be altered by hepatic and/or renal disease. These conditions inhibit drug metabolism, decrease protein synthesis, and delay elimination. In contrast, pharmacodynamic drug action is

Physiology and Pathophysiology (continued)

affected by extremes of age, hypothermia, decreased cardiac output, or the simultaneous use of other CNS depressants (eg, alcohol, illicit substances, or other sedatives).

Delayed emergence from anesthesia may also be caused by metabolic aberrations such as hypoglycemia, severe hyperglycemia, and electrolyte imbalances. A serum glucose level of less than 50 mg/dL correlates with altered level of consciousness. A high serum glucose level (eg, > 600 mg/dL) may lead to diabetic ketoacidosis, dehydration, and coma. Electrolyte abnormalities may affect central nervous, cardiovascular, respiratory, and musculoskeletal systems causing hypoventilation, altered circulation, hypoxemia, hypercarbia, acidosis, and delayed awakening.

Neurologic injury resulting in global or focal ischemic events can result in delayed emergence. Events that cause neurologic injury include cerebral trauma, cerebrovascular accident, embolic phenomena (eg, thrombus, air, or fat), increased intracranial pressure, and hematoma formation (subdural or epidural). Cerebral hypoxia and/or increased cerebral metabolic rate of oxygen consumption may also lead to neurologic damage and decreased level of consciousness.

Signs and Symptoms

Respiratory
- Altered respiratory pattern
- Hypercarbia
- Hypoxia

Cardiovascular
- Extreme hypertension
- Hypotension
- Myocardial ischemia and/or infarction

Neurologic
- Absent response to verbal or painful stimulus
- Altered level of consciousness
- Constricted, dilated, and/or nonreactive pupils

Signs and Symptoms (continued)

Neurologic
- Cushing triad
  - o Bradycardia
  - o Hypertension
  - o Irregular respiration
- Dysconjugate gaze
- Increased intracranial pressure
- Loss of somatosensory and/or motor evoked potentials during tumor resection
- Seizures

Musculoskeletal
- Decreased muscle tone or muscle flaccidity

Metabolic
- Decreased core temperature (< 35°C)
- Blood glucose level < 50 mg/dL or > 600 mg/dL
- Electrolyte abnormalities

Differential Diagnosis

Respiratory
- Airway obstruction (see Chapter 4)
- Hypercarbia (see Chapter 19)
- Hypoxia (see Chapter 24)

Cardiovascular
- Hypotension (see Chapter 22)
- Myocardial ischemia and/or infarction (see Chapter 28)

Neurologic
- Central anticholinergic syndrome
- Cerebral vascular accident
- History of cognitive (eg, dementia) or psychiatric disorders

- Hydrocephalus
- Hypoperfusion (eg, hypoxia, emboli, thrombus, shock)
- Increased intracranial pressure (eg, cerebral trauma, subdural or epidural hematoma, diffuse axonal damage)
- Neurologic surgery (eg, tumor excision)
- Postoperative cognitive dysfunction
- Seizure (eg, postictal state)

Renal
- Acute or chronic renal disease with decreased drug clearance

Differential Diagnosis (continued)

Hepatic
- Hepatitis or other hepatic disease causing decreased drug clearance

Endocrine
- Adrenal insufficiency
- Hypothyroidism

Musculoskeletal
- Neuromuscular disorders (eg, myasthenia gravis, multiple sclerosis, or Guillain-Barré syndrome)

Pharmacologic
- Prolonged effect of medications:
  1. Opioids
  2. Muscle relaxants
  3. Inhalation anesthetics
  4. Nitrous oxide
  5. Benzodiazepines
  6. Induction anesthetic agents
  7. Local anesthetic toxicity
  8. Tertiary anticholinergics (eg, scopolamine)
  9. Illicit drugs (eg, marijuana, heroin)
  10. Alcohol intoxication

Other Considerations
- Electrolyte abnormalities:
  1. Hyponatremia
  2. Hypocalcemia
  3. Hypermagnesemia
- Hyperglycemia, severe
- Hypoglycemia
- Hypothermia (see Chapter 23)
- Pseudocholinesterase deficiency
- Shock states (see Chapter 34)
- Traumatic injury

Suggested Readings

McClain DA. Delayed emergence. In: Atlee J, ed. *Complications in Anesthesia.* 2nd ed. Philadelphia, PA: Saunders Elsevier; 2007: 885-887.

Odom-Forren J. Postanesthesia recovery. In: Nagelhout JJ, Plaus KL, eds. *Nurse Anesthesia.* 4th ed. St Louis, MO: Saunders Elsevier; 2010:1218-1238.

Welliver MD. Intracranial tumor debulking. In: Elisha S, ed. *Case Studies in Nurse Anesthesia.* Sudbury, MA: Jones & Bartlett; 2011: 325-338.

Chapter 13
Difficult Airway Management

Treatment

General Considerations and Treatments

- Conduct a thorough airway assessment and consider factors that may indicate the following (see Table 13.1):
  - Difficult mask ventilation
  - Difficult laryngoscopy and intubation
  - Difficult supralaryngeal airway use and/or placement
  - Difficult cricothyrotomy placement
- Follow recommendations per the ASA difficult airway algorithm.
- Obtain and review previous anesthetic records to assess the potential for difficult ventilation and/or intubation.
- Formulate alternative plans in case difficult ventilation or intubation occurs.
- Have airway adjuncts available (see Table 13.2).
- Provide adequate preoxygenation.
- Achieve an ideal sniffing position.
- Consider administering an antisialagogue.
- Consider emergency cricothyrotomy or tracheotomy if unable to intubate and ventilate.

Anticipated Difficult Airway

- Call for assistance.
- Consider an awake fiberoptic intubation with spontaneous ventilation.

Treatment (continued)

- Consider an awake video laryngoscopy with spontaneous ventilation.
- Anesthetize the airway using local anesthesia (topical, infiltration, and/or field block).
- Titrate anesthetic medications as needed for patient to tolerate airway procedure and to maintain spontaneous respiration.

Unanticipated Difficult Airway
- Call for help.
- Maintain spontaneous ventilation.
- If muscle relaxant has already been administered, provide mask ventilation and consider use of an oropharyngeal airway.
- If ventilation by mask is inadequate, place an LMA for ventilation.
- *If ventilation is adequate,* consider use of an airway adjunct for intubation (see Table 13.2).
- Limit direct and/or video laryngoscopy (2-3 attempts).
- *If ventilation is inadequate, intubation is unsuccessful, and hypoxia exists,* consider emergency cricothyrotomy or tracheotomy.

Physiology and Pathophysiology

Difficult airway management can result in inadequate ventilation and/or intubation, oropharyngeal trauma, hypoxemia, hypercarbia, acidosis, and death. A difficult airway may be presumed if the patient has a history of difficult ventilation and/or intubation; if physical assessment of the head, neck, and oropharynx indicates the potential for difficulty; or if problems arise (eg, emergencies outside the OR, trauma, vomiting).

Physiology and Pathophysiology (continued)

A comprehensive preoperative airway assessment should include evaluation of the airway anatomy and other characteristics that influence mask ventilation, laryngoscopy, intubation, placement of a supralaryngeal device, and/or cricothyrotomy. Table 13.1 lists indications, signs, symptoms, and considerations for patients who may be at an increased risk for a difficult airway. The main objective during difficult airway management is to maintain ventilation and oxygenation. A list of difficult airway adjuncts is included in Table 13.2, and the adjuncts of choice should be immediately available in the OR.

Table 13.1. Indications, Signs, Symptoms, and Considerations for Patients at Risk for a Difficult Airway

Assessment	Signs and/or symptoms	Considerations
Difficult mask ventilation	Beard Edentulous Redundant airway tissue Mass on the face or neck Decreased cervical range of motion Wheezing Stridor History of obstructive sleep apnea Snoring Altered mandibular or maxillary anatomy Vomiting Blood or excessive secretions in the airway Foreign body in the airway Increased PIP Obesity Pregnancy	Enlarged upper and lower airway mass or a gravid uterus may cause altered ventilation by way of increased PIP and increased pressure on the diaphragm (consider raising head of bed). Use of muscle relaxants in the presence of an upper or lower airway mass may lead to an inability to ventilate and/or intubate (consider changing the patient position). Increased PIP may be a result of a foreign body, bronchospasm, ARDS, pulmonary infection, and/or pulmonary edema. Initial proper patient positioning can aid in effective mask ventilation.

Abbreviations: PIP, peak inspiratory pressure; ARDS, acute respiratory distress syndrome.

Table 13.1. Indications, Signs, Symptoms, and Considerations for Patients at Risk for a Difficult Airway (continued)

Assessment	Signs and/or symptoms	Considerations
Difficult laryngoscopy and/or intubation	Altered airway anatomy Mandibular hypoplasia Large tongue Short neck Increased neck circumference > 43 cm at the level of the thyroid cartilage Decreased cervical range of motion Prominent incisors Dental abnormalities (loose teeth) Mouth opening < 3 finger breadths Temporomandibular joint dysfunction Thyromental distance < 3 finger breadths Thyrohyoid distance < 2 finger breadths (anterior larynx) Mallampati class 3 or 4 Poor view of the glottis (Cormack-Lehane grade 3 or 4) Upper airway mass Goiter Vomiting Blood or excessive secretions in the airway Pregnancy Obesity	Scarring, masses, blood, vomit, excessive mucus, burns, or trauma could distort visualization during direct laryngoscopy or video laryngoscopy. Upper airway anatomy can be altered in a pregnant patient because of swelling of soft tissue. Muffled or hoarse voice, difficulty swallowing, stridor, and/or dyspnea are indications of upper airway obstruction. Conservative administration of sedatives in the presence of an upper airway obstruction or identified difficult laryngoscopy is prudent.
Difficult placement and ventilation using a supraglottic device	Mouth opening < 3 finger breadths Temporomandibular joint dysfunction Prominent incisors Dental abnormalities (loose teeth) Airway obstruction above or below the larynx Distorted airway anatomy Angioedema Decreased cervical range of motion Increased PIP	Upper airway masses, swelling, foreign bodies, or redundant tissue may compromise the seal of the supraglottic device. Increased PIP may be a result of a foreign body, bronchospasm, ARDS, pulmonary infection, and/or pulmonary edema resulting in difficult ventilation.
Difficult cricothyrotomy or surgical tracheotomy	Scarring of the larynx or neck (eg, surgery, radiation) Neck hematoma or mass (eg, abscess, tumor) Short neck Goiter Obesity Subcutaneous emphysema Decreased cervical range of motion	The location of a possible cricothyrotomy or tracheotomy should be identified during the preoperative airway assessment. Cricothyrotomy is reserved for emergency situations. Equipment for cricothyrotomy should be prepared before airway manipulation.

Abbreviations: PIP, peak inspiratory pressure; ARDS, acute respiratory distress syndrome.

Table 13.2. Difficult Airway Adjuncts

Airway device	Indications and considerations
Standard laryngoscope with multiple blades (straight, curved, Flex Tip Macintosh blades)	Difficult laryngoscopy and/or intubation Difficult use of a supraglottic device Consider straight blade for an elongated epiglottis. Consider curved blade for a large tongue. Flex Tip blade bends 70° further, depressing the hyoepiglottic ligament in the vallecula to provide additional lift to the epiglottis. Pregnancy
Fiberoptic bronchoscope	Anticipated difficult laryngoscopy and/or intubation Awake ETT placement (Consider antisialagogue, local anesthesia, and sedation.) Mallampati class 4 Decreased cervical range of motion (eg, arthritis, halo traction device) Restricted mouth opening Decreased thyromental and/or thyrohyoid distance (anterior larynx) Mandibular hypoplasia Upper airway obstructions Visual confirmation of ETT placement Use requires experience. Excessive blood and/or secretions can obstruct view.
Video laryngoscope (Glidescope, McGrath, Karl Storz C-MAC)	Anticipated and/or unanticipated difficult laryngoscopy and/or intubation Awake or asleep ETT placement Mallampati class III or IV Cormack-Lehane grade 3 or 4 Decreased cervical range of motion (eg, arthritis, halo traction device) Decreased mouth opening Decreased thyromental and/or thyrohyoid distance (anterior larynx) Mandibular hypoplasia Head and facial trauma Visual confirmation of ETT placement Out-of-OR emergency airway management Excessive blood and/or secretions can obstruct view.
Supraglottic devices (LMA Classic, LMA Supreme, Ambu LMA, CobraPLA, PAXpress, Cookgas ILA)	Difficult laryngoscopy and/or intubation Rescue ventilation when mask ventilation is inadequate

Abbreviations: ETT, endotracheal tube; OR, operating room.

Table 13.2. Difficult Airway Adjuncts (continued)

Airway device	Indications and considerations
Intubating LMA (Fastrach, C-Trach)	Difficult mask ventilation Anticipated/unanticipated difficult laryngoscopy and/or intubation Decreased cervical range of motion Decreased thyromental and/or thyrohyoid distance (anterior larynx) Mandibular hypoplasia Head and facial trauma Out-of-OR emergency airway management May consider using fiberoptic bronchoscope through LMA to visualize ETT placement
Eschmann stylet (gum elastic bougie)	Difficult intubation Cormack-Lehane grade 2, 3, or 4 Requires minimal training.
Lighted stylet (Laerdal Trachlight)	Difficult laryngoscopy and/or intubation Restricted mouth opening Decreased cervical range of motion Use requires experience.
Rigid and semirigid fiberoptic stylets (Shikani optical stylet, Levitan "First Pass Success" scope, Bonfils Retromolar Intubation Fiberscope, Rigid Intubating Fiberoptic Laryngoscope)	Difficult laryngoscopy and/or intubation Decreased cervical range of motion Restricted mouth opening Decreased thyromental and/or thyrohyoid distance (anterior larynx) Excessive blood and/or secretions can obstruct view.
Optically enhanced laryngoscopes (Airtraq)	Difficult laryngoscopy and/or intubation Decreased cervical range of motion Restricted mouth opening Decreased thyromental and/or thyrohyoid distance (anterior larynx) Excessive blood and/or secretions can obstruct view.
Esophageal tracheal tube (Combitube, King LT Airway, Rusch EasyTube)	Difficult mask ventilation Difficult laryngoscopy and/or intubation Difficult placement of a supralaryngeal device Use can be considered during preparation for a cricothyrotomy.
Retrograde wire	Difficult laryngoscopy and/or intubation Trauma to supralaryngeal structures
Cricothyrotomy	Cannot intubate, cannot ventilate Emergency airway management Trauma to supralaryngeal structures Standard intubation is deemed impossible.

Abbreviations: ETT, endotracheal tube; OR, operating room.

Signs and Symptoms

- See Table 13.1.
- Any factor that can lead to the following:
    1. Difficult mask ventilation
    2. Difficult laryngoscopy and intubation
    3. Difficult placement or ventilation with a supraglottic device
    4. Difficult cricothyrotomy or surgical tracheotomy

Differential Diagnosis

Respiratory
- Airway obstruction (see Chapter 4)
- Airway trauma
- Altered airway anatomy (tumors, goiters, scarring)
- Angioedema
- Laryngospasm (see Chapter 25)
- Ludwig angina
- Obstructive sleep apnea
- Pneumothorax or tension pneumothorax (see Chapter 31)
- Pulmonary edema
- Smoke inhalation
- Upper or lower airway infection (epiglottitis, pneumonia)

Musculoskeletal
- Ankylosing spondylitis
- Craniofacial abnormalities (eg, Down syndrome, Treacher-Collins syndrome, Pierre Robin syndrome)
- Mandibular hypoplasia
- Obesity
- Rheumatoid arthritis

Other Considerations
- Emergency airway management outside the OR (eg, ED, ICU)
- Pregnancy
- Radiation therapy to the airway
- Trauma

Suggested Readings

American Society of Anesthesiologists Task Force on Management of the Difficult Airway. Practice guidelines for management of the difficult airway: an updated report. *Anesthesiology*. 2003;98(5): 1269-1277.

Chipas A, Ellis WE. Airway management. In: Nagelhout JJ, Plaus KL, eds. *Nurse Anesthesia*. 4th ed. St Louis, MO: Saunders Elsevier; 2010: 441-464.

Murphy MF, Walls RM. Identification of the difficult and failed airway. In: Walls RM, Murphy MF, eds. *Manual of Emergency Airway Management*. 3rd ed. Philadelphia, PA: Lippincott Williams & Wilkins; 2008:81-93.

Chapter 14
Disseminated Intravascular Coagulation

Treatment

- Treat underlying pathological state.
- Administer blood products based on clinical and laboratory assessment.
- Massive transfusion protocol using one of the following target ratios for blood products to maintain appropriate hemoglobin concentration and coagulation status:
  - 1 U PRBC + 1 U FFP + 1 platelet concentrate (ie, equal to 1 pooled unit)
  - 4 U PRBC + 4 U FFP + 1 platelet apheresis (ie, equal to 4-6 pooled units)
- Administer recombinant activated factor VII and cryoprecipitate when appropriate.
- Administer supportive measures as needed:
  - Airway management
  - Invasive monitoring (eg, arterial line, CVP)
  - Central venous access
  - Vasopressor medication(s)
  - Inotropic medication(s)
- Administer antibiotic medication(s) when appropriate.
- Avoid lethal triad:
  - Acidosis
  - Hypothermia
  - Coagulopathy
- Monitor laboratory values (eg, CBC, platelet count, PT/PTT/INR, fibrinogen, electrolytes, ABG, D-dimer).

Physiology and Pathophysiology

DIC is a symptom of an underlying pathological process capable of activating systemic inflammation and coagulation.

Conditions that predispose patients to DIC include the following:

- Sepsis
- Massive trauma and shock states
- Obstetric complications (eg, retained placental fragments, amniotic fluid embolism)
- Malignant disease
- Vascular disease
- Embolic event
- Immune-mediated disorders
- Systemic toxins
- Primary organ failure

Therefore, treatment for DIC must focus on identifying and correcting the underlying pathological state. The clinical presentation of DIC may include thrombosis, hemorrhage, or both. Systemic activation of coagulation results in (1) intravascular deposition of fibrin, (2) thrombotic microangiopathy, (3) compromised blood supply to organs, and (4) multiorgan system failure. Systemic activation of coagulation also promotes the use and subsequent depletion of platelets and coagulation factors (eg, consumptive coagulopathy), which may induce severe bleeding from multiple sites.

Signs and Symptoms

Respiratory
- Dyspnea
- Hypoxia
- Tachypnea

Cardiovascular
- Cardiac dysrhythmias
- Hemodynamic instability

Neurologic
- Altered level of consciousness

Signs and Symptoms (continued)

Hematologic
- Hemorrhage
  1. Bleeding from mucous membranes and skin (eg, petechiae and ecchymosis)
  2. Bleeding from surgical sites, wounds, invasive monitor sites, or venipuncture sites
- Laboratory abnormalities
  1. Elevated fibrin degradation products (eg, D-dimer immunoassay)
  2. Moderate to severe antithrombin deficiency
  3. Moderate to severe hypofibrinogenemia
  4. Moderate to severe thrombocytopenia
  5. Prolonged clotting time (eg, prothrombin time and activated partial thromboplastin time)
- Thrombosis
  1. Peripheral acrocyanosis
  2. Pregangrenous changes to peripheral tissue (eg, hands, feet, genitalia, and nose)
  3. Purpura fulminans

Other Considerations
- Multiorgan system failure
  o Elevated serum markers (eg, hepatic, renal, and cardiac)

Differential Diagnosis

Respiratory
- ARDS
- TRALI (see Chapter 37)

Cardiovascular
- Fat embolism (see Chapter 17)
- Hypovolemia
- Vascular disease
  1. Kasabach-Merritt syndrome (eg, giant hemangioma)
  2. Large vessel aneurysm (eg, aortic aneurysm)

Neurologic
- Traumatic brain injury

Hematologic
- Hemolytic transfusion reaction
- Massive transfusion
- Thrombotic thrombocytopenic purpura

75

Differential Diagnosis (continued)

Gastrointestinal
- Fulminant hepatic failure

Pharmacologic
- Illicit drug use (eg, metham-phetamine overdose)

Other Considerations
- Immune-mediated disorders
  1. Adult Still disease
  2. Allergic reactions
  3. Lupus erythematosus
  4. Transplant rejection
- Malignant disease
  1. Cytotoxic chemotherapy
  2. Myeloproliferative malig-nancy (eg, acute promy-elocytic leukemia)
  3. Pancreatic carcinoma
  4. Solid tumors (eg, meta-static adenocarcinoma)
  5. Trousseau syndrome (eg, chronic compensated DIC)
  6. Tumor lysis syndrome
- Massive trauma and shock states (eg, extensive burns)

- Obstetrical complications
  1. Amniotic fluid embolism (see Chapter 17)
  2. HELLP syndrome
  3. Placenta previa
  4. Placental abruption
  5. Retained dead fetus or products of conception syndrome
  6. Septic miscarriage or abortion
- Sepsis
  1. Fungal
  2. Gram-negative and gram-positive bacterial
  3. Helminthic
  4. Malarial
  5. Protozoan
  6. Rocky Mountain spotted fever
  7. Viral
- Systemic toxins (eg, snake venom)

Suggested Readings

D'Angelo MR, Dutton RP. Management of trauma-induced coagulopathy: trends and practices. *AANA J.* 2010;78(1):35-40.

Franco JA. Hematology and anesthesia. In: Nagelhout JJ, Plaus KL, eds. *Nurse Anesthesia.* 4th ed. St Louis, MO: Saunders Elsevier; 2010: 842-861.

Labelle CA, Kitchens, CS. Disseminated intravascular coagulation: treat the cause, not the lab values. *Cleve Clin J Med.* 2005;72(5): 377-397.

Shaz BH, Dente CJ, Harris RS, MacLeod JB, Hillyer CD. Transfusion management of trauma patients. *Anesth Analg.* 2009;108(6):1760-1768.

Chapter 15
Electrical Power Failure

Treatment

- Call for help.
- Ensure adequate airway, breathing, and circulation.
  - If anesthesia machine is not functioning, use bag-valve device connected to auxiliary flowmeter or oxygen tank to ventilate patient.
  - Obtain basic vital signs via transport monitor or traditional means (eg, sphygmomanometer, manual assessment of pulse, auscultation of breath sounds).
  - Assess backup power and battery life of anesthesia machine.
- For a patient who is anesthetized, ensure the delivery of anesthesia via TIVA.
- Use battery-powered electrical devices and emergency equipment (eg, flashlight, airway equipment, and transport monitor) to assess the patient and provide anesthesia.
- Determine the estimated time for the return of power.
- Discuss with the surgical team the necessity to continue or discontinue the surgical procedure.
- Assess the feasibility of transferring the patient to a location with power.

Physiology and Pathophysiology

The electrical power to an OR originates from the electrical company or hospital emergency generator. The electrical current then passes through 2 isolated power systems within the hospital via the isolation transformer. Electrical power is then transferred to the standard and emergency electrical outlets located throughout the hospital (including ORs). Finally, electricity is provided to electrical devices that are plugged into these electrical outlets. A disruption in the circuit of electrical power at any stage of this process will cause partial or total electrical power failure to an OR. Care for the patient during an electrical power failure includes the following:

- Ensuring the adequacy of airway patency, breathing, and circulation
- Providing appropriate patient monitoring (eg, heart rate, heart rhythm, blood pressure, oxygenation)
- Providing appropriate anesthesia management

Signs and Symptoms

Cessation of function in equipment that is electrically powered:

- Anesthesia equipment malfunction (see Chapter 6)
  - Advanced airway equipment (eg, video laryngoscope)
  - Anesthesia machine (eg, ventilator and desflurane vaporizer)
  - Medication dispensing machine (Pyxis)
  - Standard and invasive monitoring devices
- OR equipment malfunction
  - Ambient and surgical lighting
  - Cardiopulmonary bypass equipment
  - Fluid and warming devices
  - OR bed
  - Surgical instruments (eg, electrocautery and laparoscopy equipment)

Differential Diagnosis

- Anesthesia machine alarms indicating power failure
- Electrocution (microshock or macroshock)
- Extreme weather conditions
- Failure of electrical equipment
- Failure of electrical outlets
- Failure of emergency generator
- Failure of isolation transformer
- Internal or external hospital construction
- Natural disaster (eg, fire, earthquake)

Suggested Readings

Barker SJ, Doyle DJ. Electrical safety in the operating room: dry versus wet [editorial]. *Anesth Analg*. 2010;110(6):1517-1518.

Carpenter T, Robinson ST. Case reports: response to a partial power failure in the operating room. *Anesth Analg*. 2010;110(6):1644-1646.

Eichhorn JH, Hessel EA Jr. Electrical power failure in the operating room: a neglected topic in anesthesia safety [editorial]. *Anesth Analg*. 2010;110(6):1519-1521.

Chapter 16
Electrolyte Abnormalities

Treatment

- Manage CNS, cardiac, and neuromuscular manifestations.
- Treat underlying pathological cause.
- Monitor fluid status (eg, urinary catheter, CVP), and manage appropriately.
- Monitor acid-base status (eg, ABG analysis), and manage appropriately.
- Consider electrolyte-specific replacement for total body deficits. (See Table 16.1 for specific electrolyte imbalances and treatment.)
- Administer supportive measures as needed:
    - Cardiac resuscitation per American Heart Association ACLS or PALS protocol as necessary
    - Invasive monitoring (eg, arterial line, CVP)
    - Central venous access
    - Vasopressor medication(s)
    - Inotropic medication(s)
    - Antidysrhythmic medication(s)

Physiology and Pathophysiology

Intracellular and extracellular concentrations of electrolytes (eg, sodium, potassium, calcium, and magnesium) are essential for maintaining concentration gradients across cellular membranes. Electrolyte imbalances produce alterations in cellular electrophysiology (eg, resting membrane potential, threshold potential, action potential, and neurotransmission). Thus, perioperative alterations in electrolyte content and distribution can produce multiorgan system dysfunction. The treatment of electrolyte imbalances should be based on identifying and treating the underlying pathological state.

Electrolyte content and distribution within the body are influenced by numerous factors, including (1) fluid status (total body water content and distribution), (2) acid-base status, and (3) endocrine function (hypothalamus, pituitary gland, thyroid gland, parathyroid glands, adrenal cortex, and kidney). Electrolyte imbalances are often a reflection of at least 1 of these factors. The severity of an electrolyte imbalance is dependent on (1) etiology, (2) onset and duration (acute or chronic presentation), (3) absolute electrolyte imbalance, and (4) effects on organ function (CNS, cardiac, and neuromuscular).

Signs and Symptoms

Respiratory
- Dyspnea
- Laryngospasm (see Chapter 25)
- Tachypnea

Cardiovascular
- Altered myocardial contractility
- Cardiac conduction abnormalities
- Dysrhythmias
- Hypertension
- Hypotension
- Myocardial infarction or ischemia

Neurologic
- Altered deep tendon reflexes
- Altered level of consciousness
- Delayed emergence from anesthesia

Signs and Symptoms (continued)

Neurologic
- Paresthesias
- Seizures

Musculoskeletal
- Skeletal muscle tetany
- Skeletal muscle weakness

Differential Diagnosis

- See Table 16.1 for symptoms, differential diagnosis, and treatment of specific electrolyte imbalances.

Table 16.1. Electrolyte Imbalances: Symptoms, Differential Diagnosis, and Treatment

	Sodium		Potassium	
	Hyponatremia	**Hypernatremia**	**Hypokalemia**	**Hyperkale**
Signs and symptoms	Serum concentration < 135 mEq/L Altered level of consciousness Brainstem herniation Cerebral edema Increased ICP Respiratory arrest Seizures Cardiac dysrhythmias	Serum concentration > 145 mEq/L Ascites Decreased urine output Hypotension and tachycardia Increased BUN and creatinine levels Increased urine specific gravity Pleural effusion	Serum concentration < 3.5 mEq/L Cardiac dysrhythmias (U wave, flattened or inverted T wave) Digoxin toxicity Orthostatic hypotension Skeletal muscle weakness	Serum concentra > 5.5 mEq/L Cardiac dysrhyth (peaked T wave prolonged P-R absent P wave, QRS, and ventr arrhythmias) Skeletal muscle w
Differential diagnosis	Addison disease Corticosteroid depletion Excess absorption of irrigation solutions (TURP syndrome) Gastrointestinal loss Heart, liver, and renal failure Hypoadrenalism Hypothyroidism Overhydration and/or excess water ingestion SIADH Thiazide diuretics	Corticosteroid excess Cushing disease Dehydration and/ or decreased water ingestion Diabetes insipidus Hyperventilation Osmotic diuretics Renal failure (impaired sodium excretion)	Antibiotics (penicillin analogs and aminogly-cosides) Cushing disease Diuretics (thiazide and loop diuretics) Gastrointestinal loss Hyperaldosteronism Hyperglycemia Insulin overdose Mineralocorticoid and glucocorticoid drugs Respiratory/metabolic alkalosis β-adrenergic agonists	ACE inhibitors Acute and chron failure Addison disease Diuretics (spiron tone and triam Hypoaldosteron NSAIDs Respiratory or m acidosis Succinylcholine a tration followin spinal cord inju injury, and prol immobilization β-adrenergic ant
Treatment	Treat pathological cause Water restriction to < 800 mL/d Loop diuretics (furosemide) Hypertonic saline (3% or 5%), 1-2 mL/kg/h not to exceed 100 mL/h	Treat pathological cause Electrolyte free water (5% glucose in water), maximum rate of correction 0.5 mEq/L/h Potassium-sparing diuretics (spironolactone)	Treat pathological cause Potassium replacement for true deficit, maximum rate of replacement 20 mEq/h (0.2 mEq/kg/h)	Treat pathologica Calcium 10% chl (10 mL over 10 or calcium gluc Glucose and insu (5-10 U per 25-50 g of gluc Sodium bicarbon (50-150 mEq o 5-10 minutes) β_2 agonists Hyperventilation Hemodialysis

Abbreviations: ICP, intracranial pressure; BUN, blood urea nitrogen; TURP, transurethral resection of the prostate; SIADH, syndrome of inappropriate secretion of antidiuretic hormone; ACE, angiotens converting enzyme; NSAID, nonsteroidal anti-inflammatory drug.

le 16.1. Electrolyte Imbalances: Symptoms, Differential Diagnosis,
Treatment (continued)

	Calcium		Magnesium	
	Hypocalcemia	**Hypercalcemia**	**Hypomagnesemia**	**Hypermagnesemia**
and toms	Serum concentration < 4.5 mEq/L Cardiac dysrhythmias (shortened P-R interval and prolonged Q-T interval) Chvostek and/or Trousseau signs Circumoral paresthesia Hypotension Laryngospasm Seizures	Serum concentration > 5.5 mEq/L Cardiac dysrhythmias (prolonged P-R interval, shortened Q-T interval and ST segment) Digitalis toxicity Hypertension	Serum concentration < 1.5 mEq/L Altered response to muscle relaxants Cardiac dysrhythmias (torsades de pointes) Digitalis toxicity Hyperreflexia Increased deep tendon reflexes Seizures Skeletal muscle spasms	Serum concentration > 2.5 mEq/L Cardiac and respiratory arrest Coma Depressed deep tendon reflexes Hyporeflexia Sedation Skeletal muscle weakness
ntial nosis	Acute pancreatitis Decreased plasma albumin level Decreased serum magnesium level Hypertonic phosphate enemas Hypoparathyroidism Increased serum fatty acid level Renal failure Respiratory alkalosis Vitamin D deficiency	Hyperparathyroidism Immobilization Neoplastic bone metastases Sarcoidosis Vitamin D toxicity	Chronic alcoholism Gastrointestinal loss Hyperalimentation therapy without magnesium Malabsorption syndromes	Chronic renal failure Iatrogenic (administration for pregnancy-induced hypertension and excessive use of antacids or laxatives)
nent	Treat pathological cause Calcium replacement (10% calcium gluconate 10 mL in 10 minutes) Thiazide diuretics	Treat pathological cause Hydration with normal saline Loop diuretics (furosemide) Bisphosphonates Hemodialysis Mithramycin	Treat pathological cause Magnesium replacement (magnesium sulfate 1-3g IV over 15 minutes)	Treat pathological cause Calcium administration Fluid administration Diuretics Hemodialysis

iations: ICP, intracranial pressure; BUN, blood urea nitrogen; TURP, transurethral resection of
state; SIADH, syndrome of inappropriate secretion of antidiuretic hormone; ACE, angiotensin-
:ing enzyme; NSAID, nonsteroidal anti-inflammatory drug.

Suggested Readings

Luckey AE, Parsa CJ. Fluid and electrolytes in the aged. *Arch Surg.* 2003;138(10):1055-1060.

Rassam SS, Counsell DJ. Perioperative electrolyte and fluid balance. *Cont Educ Anaesth Crit Care Pain.* 2005;5(5):157-160.

Waters E, Nishinaga AK. Fluids, electrolytes, and blood component therapy. In: Nagelhout JJ, Plaus KL, eds. *Nurse Anesthesia.* 4th ed. St Louis, MO: Saunders Elsevier; 2010:401-419.

Chapter 17
Embolism

Venous Air Embolism or Carbon Dioxide Gas Embolism
- For VAE, tell surgeon to flood the surgical field.
- For carbon dioxide gas embolism, tell the surgeon to remove the pneumoperitoneum.
- Call for help.
- Administer 100% oxygen with manual bag ventilation.
- Discontinue all anesthetic agents.
- Avoid nitrous oxide.
- Administer IV fluid bolus.
- For VAE, reposition the patient in the LLDP with the head below the level of the heart.
- For carbon dioxide gas embolism, reposition patient in the LLDP.
- Administer vasopressor(s) and/or inotropic medications.
- Insert central line and aspirate air or gas embolism.
- Consider transesophageal echocardiogram.
- Perform ACLS or PALS per American Heart Association protocol.

Pulmonary Embolism (thrombus)
- Administer 100% oxygen.
- Call for help.
- Perform endotracheal intubation if respiratory distress occurs.
- Discontinue all anesthetic agents.
- Support circulation with fluid bolus, vasopressor(s), and/or inotropic medications.
- Obtain ABG results.
- Administer PEEP to help treat hypoxia if normotension exists.

Treatment (continued)

- Obtain ventilation-perfusion scan.
- Initiate heparin anticoagulation.
- Consider pulmonary embolectomy.
- Perform ACLS or PALS per American Heart Association protocol.

Fat Embolism
- Administer 100% oxygen.
- Call for help.
- Perform endotracheal intubation if respiratory distress occurs.
- Discontinue all anesthetic agents.
- Support circulation with fluid bolus, vasopressor(s), and/or inotropic medications.
- Obtain ABG results.
- Administer PEEP to help treat hypoxia if normotension exists.
- Perform ACLS or PALS per American Heart Association protocol.

Amniotic Fluid Embolism
- Administer 100% oxygen.
- Call for help.
- Perform endotracheal intubation.
- Deliver the fetus immediately.
- Discontinue all anesthetic agents.
- Support circulation with fluid bolus, vasopressor(s), and/or inotropic medications.
- Obtain ABG results.
- Administer PEEP to help treat hypoxia if normotension exists.
- Obtain coagulation panel.
- Type and crossmatch for PRBC, FFP, platelets.
- Consider uterotonic agents if uterine atony is present.
- Perform ACLS or PALS per American Heart Association protocol.

Physiology and Pathophysiology

Physiological manifestations of specific causes of an embolism (eg, venous air, carbon dioxide, thrombus, fat, or amniotic fluid) result in inadequate blood flow through the heart and pulmonary vasculature. These causes are listed in Table 17.1. The inherent decrease in intracardiac and pulmonary blood flow causes (1) an increase in physiological dead space, (2) ventilation and/or perfusion mismatch, (3) hypoxemia and/or hypercarbia, and (4) decreased stroke volume.

Venous Air Embolism
Venous air embolism is caused by ambient air entrained into an open vein. This most commonly occurs when the surgical site is positioned above the level of the heart (eg, sitting craniotomy or central line placement). An airlock is formed as gas congregates at the inflow tract to the right atrium. Air can also migrate into the pulmonary artery, further disrupting blood flow. The result is decreased or absent cardiac output and increased dead space ventilation, respectively. The severity of the VAE is determined by the amount of air that is absorbed and the rate of entry.

Carbon Dioxide Gas Embolism
Carbon dioxide gas embolism can occur when the carbon dioxide gas that is used during insufflation in laparoscopic procedures is entrained rapidly and in substantial amounts into the central circulation. The remaining pathophysiology is the same as the description for VAE.

Pulmonary Embolism
Pulmonary embolism is caused by the migration of a thrombus into the pulmonary vascular bed. The result is an obstruction within the pulmonary artery (ie, thrombus) that increases dead space and can cause hypoxemia, decreased stroke volume, and cardiac arrest.

Physiology and Pathophysiology (continued)

Fat Embolism

Fat embolism is frequently associated with pelvic and long bone fractures that occur during trauma. When venous pressure is low, fat emboli can migrate into a lacerated vein and then into systemic circulation causing cerebrovascular and/or pulmonary artery obstruction. However, fat embolus syndrome can occur during routine surgical procedures such as hip replacement. It is thought that as the fat emboli are broken down in the lungs, free fatty acids are released, which can cause interstitial hemorrhaging and pneumocyte dysfunction. The remaining pathophysiology is the same as the description for pulmonary embolism.

Amniotic Fluid Embolism

Amniotic fluid embolism and its associated pathophysiology are poorly understood. It has been theorized that amniotic fluid, which under normal conditions does not enter maternal circulation, leeches into the bloodstream through endocervical veins at the placental insertion or through a laceration at a site where the uterus has been traumatized.

Pathophysiologic changes associated with amniotic fluid embolism occur in 2 phases:

Phase 1: Severe pulmonary artery vasoconstriction resulting in decreased pulmonary blood flow and hypoxemia, elevated right-sided heart pressure, decreased left ventricular preload, decreased stroke volume, and potential cardiovascular collapse.

Phase 2: Inflammatory mediator release, hemorrhage from uterine atony, and DIC.

Signs and Symptoms

Respiratory
- Decreased or absent ETCO$_2$
- Decreased oxygen saturation
- Dyspnea
- Hypercarbia
- Hypoxemia
- Rales and/or wheezing
- Respiratory arrest
- Shortness of breath
- Tachypnea

Cardiovascular
- Cardiac arrest
- Cardiac dysrhythmias
- Chest pain
- Increased CVP
- Increased pulmonary artery pressure
- Jugular venous distention
- Loss of consciousness
- Tachycardia
- See Table 17.1 for signs, symptoms, and differentiating factors for various embolic states.

Table 17.1. Signs, Symptoms, and Differentiating Factors for Various Types of Emboli

	Air or gas	**Amniotic**	**Pulmonary**	**Fat**
Specific signs and symptoms	Mill wheel murmur Bubbles in heart on transesophageal echocardiography End-tidal nitrogen on mass spectrometry (air embolism only) Subcutaneous emphysema (CO$_2$ embolism only)	Bleeding DIC	Hemoptysis	Petechiae DIC Anemia Low platelets Cor pulmonale
Differentiating factors	Air: Occurs in any procedure when open vein is positioned higher than the heart CO$_2$: Occurs during laparoscopic procedures	Associated with labor and delivery	Associated with deep vein thrombosis Diagnosis: ventilation-perfusion scan	Associated with pelvic and long bone fractures

Abbreviations: CO$_2$, carbon dioxide; DIC, disseminated intravascular coagulation.

Differential Diagnosis

Respiratory
- Bronchospasm
  (see Chapter 8)
- ETT obstruction
  (eg, mucous plug, kink)
- Hypercarbia (see Chapter 19)
- Hypoxia (see Chapter 24)

Cardiovascular
- Acute AV valvular
  dysfunction
- Cardiac dysrhythmias
  (see Chapter 9)

- Cardiogenic shock
  (see Chapter 34)
- Hypotension
  (see Chapter 22)
- Myocardial ischemia and/or
  infarction (see Chapter 28)
- Shock states
  (see Chapter 34)

Gastrointestinal
- Acute gastric aspiration
  (see Chapter 2)

Other Considerations
- Anaphylaxis (see Chapter 5)

Suggested Readings

Clark SL. Amniotic fluid embolism. *Clin Obstet Gynecol.* 2010;53(2): 322-328.

Elisha S. Posterior spinal reconstructive surgery. In: Elisha S, ed. *Case Studies in Nurse Anesthesia.* Sudbury, MA: Jones & Bartlett; 2011: 531-542.

Jadik S, Wissing H, Friedrich K, Beck J, Seifert V, Raabe A. A standardized protocol for the prevention of clinically relevant venous air embolism during neurosurgical interventions in the semisitting position. *Neurosurgery.* 2009;64(3):533-538.

Chapter 18
Hemorrhage (acute and chronic)

Treatment

- Treat underlying pathological state.
- Manage cardiac, pulmonary, and neurologic manifestations.
- Obtain multiple large-bore peripheral IV access and/or central venous access.
- Administer IV fluids using crystalloids, colloids, blood, and/or blood products.
- Ensure surgical management:
    - Direct pressure to wound or surgical site
    - Topical hemostatic agents (eg, Evithrom [Ethicon Inc, Somerville, NJ], Gelfoam [Baxter Healthcare Corporation, Hayward, CA; and Surgicel [Ethicon, Inc])
    - Surgical ligation or clamping of blood vessels (eg, aortic cross-clamping)
- Administer blood products based on hemoglobin and/or coagulation status.
- For massive transfusion, consider a fast-flow blood and fluid warming system (eg, level 1 infuser).
- For blood replacement during massive resuscitation effort, consider administration ratio of 1 PRBC:1 FFP:1 platelet.
- Monitor fluid, hemoglobin, electrolyte (including calcium), and acid-base results.
- Administer supportive measures when appropriate:
    - Invasive monitoring
    - Vasopressor medication(s)
    - Inotropic medication(s)
    - Antifibrinolytics (ε-aminocaproic acid and tranexamic acid)

Treatment (continued)

- o Autologous blood cell salvage (eg, intraoperative autotransfusion)
- o Cryoprecipitation
- o Factor VII
- Avoid lethal triad:
  - o Acidosis
  - o Hypothermia
  - o Coagulopathy

Physiology and Pathophysiology

The World Health Organization has defined *anemia* as a hemoglobin concentration of less than 13 g/dL for men and less than 12 g/dL for nonpregnant women. Perioperative anemia is attributed to (1) decreased erythrocyte production, (2) increased erythrocyte loss, (3) increased erythrocyte destruction, and/or (4) decreased serum hemoglobin concentration. Undiagnosed anemia is the most common hematological problem that occurs during perioperative patient management. Preoperative anemia may be a sign of an underlying pathological state or condition that may affect surgical outcome. In this instance, it is prudent to delay major elective surgery until the cause of anemia is identified, treated, and medically optimized (eg, iron supplementation or erythropoietic-stimulating agents).

Decreased perioperative hemoglobin reduces the oxygen-carrying capacity of blood and is a serious factor for morbidity and mortality, especially in patients with cardiopulmonary and neurovascular disease. Medical management of acute anemia (eg, hemorrhage)

Physiology and Pathophysiology (continued)

should attempt to (1) stop hemorrhage, (2) maintain hemodynamic stability, (3) maximize blood oxygen-carrying capacity, (4) maximize oxygen delivery to peripheral and central tissues, and (5) avoid coagulopathy. Allogeneic blood transfusion can cause (1) viral transmission, (2) bacterial contamination, (3) transfusion-related acute lung injury, (4) transfusion-related cardiac overload, and (5) acute transfusion reactions. The ASA guidelines for allogeneic blood transfusion include the following:

- Transfusion is rarely necessary when the hemoglobin concentration is greater than 10 g/dL.
- Transfusion is usually indicated when hemoglobin concentration is less than 6 g/dL.
- When the hemoglobin concentrations are between 6 g/dL and 10 g/dL, the decision to transfuse is determined by the following:
  o Evidence of organ ischemia (hypotension, dysrhythmias)
  o Actual or potential bleeding
  o Presence of risk factors that cause inadequate oxygenation (eg, decreased cardiopulmonary reserve)

Signs and Symptoms

Respiratory
- CHF
- Dyspnea
- Hemoptysis
- Hypercarbia
- Hypoxia
- Pulmonary edema
- Tachypnea

Cardiovascular
- Angina pectoris
- Arterial waveform amplitude variation with respiration
- Decreased peripheral and/or central pulses
- Dysrhythmias
- Frank bleeding (eg, hemorrhage)

Signs and Symptoms (continued)

- Hypotension
- Low and/or narrow pulse pressure
- Low CVP
- Low left ventricular end-diastolic pressure
- Myocardial infarction or ischemia
- Orthostatic hypotension
- Palpitations
- Pulse oximetry plethysmographic waveform amplitude variation with respiration
- Systemic hypotension
- Tachycardia

Neurologic
- Altered level or loss of consciousness
- Confusion
- Fatigue
- Restlessness

Renal
- Hematuria
- Oliguria

Hematologic
- Hemoglobin concentration of less than 13 g/dL for men and less than 12 g/dL for nonpregnant women

Gastrointestinal
- Hematemesis
- Hematochezia
- Hepatosplenomegaly
- Melena

Musculoskeletal
- Bone pain

Other Considerations
- Integumentary
  1. Pallor of skin and mucous membranes
  2. Petechiae
  3. Purpura
- Physical examination
  1. Lymphadenopathy
  2. Metabolic acidosis (eg, lactic acidosis)
  3. Menstrual blood loss

Differential Diagnosis

Respiratory
- Cystic and cavitary pulmonary disease (eg, tuberculosis)
- Goodpasture syndrome
- Lung cancer
- Pulmonary embolus

Differential Diagnosis (continued)

Cardiovascular
- CHF
- Hypotension (see Chapter 22)
- Retroperitoneal bleeding (eg, discoloration of flank region)
- Rupture of major blood vessels from trauma
- Ruptured aneurysm (aortic or cerebral)

Renal
- Renal disease
- Renal trauma

Endocrine
- Acute adrenal crises (see Chapter 1)
- Hypoadrenalism
- Hypopituitarism
- Hypothyroidism

Hematologic
- Aplastic anemia (Fanconi or Diamond-Blackfan syndrome)
- Hemolytic anemia
  - Autoantibody transfusion reaction
  - Autoimmune-mediated disease
  - DIC
  - Erythrocyte cell membrane disorder (hereditary spherocytosis or elliptocytosis)
  - Erythrocyte enzymopathy (eg, glucose-6-phosphate dehydrogenase deficiency)
  - Erythrocyte pyruvate kinase deficiency
  - Hemoglobin Hammersmith
  - Hemolytic uremic syndrome
  - Infection-mediated disease
  - Microangiopathic hemolytic anemia
  - Paroxysmal nocturnal hemoglobinuria
  - Sickle cell disease
  - Thrombotic thrombocytopenic purpura
- Iron deficiency anemia
- Megaloblastic anemia
  - Folate deficiency
  - Vitamin B_{12} deficiency
- Myeloproliferative disorder
- Thalassemia

Gastrointestinal
- Colon cancer
- Colonic diverticula or diverticulitis
- Esophageal varices
- Esophagogastric mucosal laceration (eg, Mallory-Weiss syndrome)
- Gastric and duodenal ulcers
- Gastritis
- Liver disease
- Liver trauma

Differential Diagnosis (continued)

Pharmacologic

- Alcohol
- Anticonvulsants
- Antithrombotic medication (eg, antiplatelet, anticoagulant, or fibrinolytic)
- Chemotherapy
- Exogenous allergens (eg, penicillin allergy)
- Methemoglobinemia
- Sulfhemoglobinemia

Other Considerations

- Anemia of chronic disease
  - Hypersplenism
  - Metastatic cancer
- Mechanical origin
  - Disconnected intra-arterial device (eg, arterial line, aortic cannula, and intra-aortic balloon catheter)

- Obstetric or gynecologic origin
  - Abruptio placenta
  - Obstetric hemorrhage due to uterine atony (see Chapter 29)
  - Placenta accreta, increta, or percreta
  - Placenta previa
  - Ruptured ectopic pregnancy
  - Ruptured ovarian cyst
  - Uterine rupture
- Traumatic injury
  - Extensive burn injury
  - Laceration(s)
  - Penetrating injury (eg, gunshot wounds, stab wounds, and projectiles)

Suggested Readings

American Society of Anesthesiologists Task Force on Perioperative Blood Transfusion and Adjuvant Therapies. Practice guidelines for perioperative blood transfusion and adjuvant therapies: an updated report. *Anesthesiology.* 2006;105(1):198-208.

Barton CR, Radesic BP. Trauma anesthesia. In: Nagelhout JJ, Plaus KL, eds. *Nurse Anesthesia.* 4th ed. St Louis, MO: Saunders Elsevier; 2010:875-891.

Patel MS, Carson JL. Anemia in the preoperative patient. *Anesthesiol Clin.* 2009;27(4):751-760.

Chapter 19
Hypercarbia

- Maintain airway, breathing, and circulation.
- Provide F_{IO_2} at 100%.
- Assess the presence or absence of abnormal breath sounds.
- Assess signs and symptoms associated with hypercarbia.
- For a spontaneously breathing anesthetized patient:
  - Assist ventilation with bag-valve-mask device.
  - Apply noxious stimuli (eg, chin lift, jaw thrust).
  - Decrease anesthetic depth.
  - Consider reversal of narcotics (eg, naloxone).
  - Consider reversal of benzodiazepines (eg, flumazenil).
- For a mechanically ventilated patient receiving general anesthesia:
  - Confirm correct placement of airway management device (LMA or ETT).
  - Use manual ventilation mode and assist ventilation to increase minute ventilation (respiratory rate and/or tidal volume).
- Obtain ABG results.
- Identify and treat definitive cause(s).

Physiology and Pathophysiology

Carbon dioxide is a natural by-product of cellular metabolism. *Hypercarbia* is defined as a Pa_{CO_2} greater than 45 mm Hg and occurs because of increased production and/or decreased elimination of carbon dioxide. Central chemoreceptors located in the ventrolateral medulla and peripheral chemoreceptors located in the aortic and carotid bodies are sensitive to hydrogen ions and carbon dioxide. The physiological response to hypercarbia includes SNS hyperactivity, which causes tachycardia, tachypnea, and hypertension. Excessive carbon dioxide in the blood will react with water to produce an abundance of hydrogen ions, as shown in Equation 19.1. If the amount of carbon dioxide is extreme, and the respiratory and renal systems cannot compensate to substantially decrease hydrogen ion concentrations, acidosis will occur.

Equation 19.1. Formation of Hydrogen Ions From CO_2 Reaction With H_2O

$$CO_2 + H_2O \longleftrightarrow H_2CO_3 \longleftrightarrow H^+ + HCO_3^-$$

Signs and Symptoms

Respiratory
- Absent or diminished breath sounds
- Hypertension
- Increased $ETCO_2$
- Increased Pa_{CO_2}
- Pulmonary infiltrates on chest radiograph
- Rales
- Respiratory acidosis
- Spontaneous respirations during manual ventilation in partially paralyzed and/or adequately anesthetized patient
- Tachypnea
- Wheezes

Signs and Symptoms (continued)

Cardiovascular
- Cardiac arrest
- Dysrhythmias
- Tachycardia

Other Considerations
- Altered level of consciousness
- Hyperkalemia
- Hyperthermia

Differential Diagnosis

Respiratory
- Acute gastric aspiration (see Chapter 2)
- ARDS
- Airway fire (see Chapter 3)
- Airway obstruction (see Chapter 4)
- Bronchospasm (see Chapter 8)
- COPD
- Endobronchial intubation
- Fractured ribs, pulmonary contusion, and/or diaphragmatic rupture
- Hypoventilation
- Metastatic lung disease
- Pneumothorax and/or tension pneumothorax (see Chapter 31)
- Positioning (reverse Trendelenburg, lithotomy)
- Postoperative pain during respiration
- Pulmonary edema
- Pulmonary embolism (see Chapter 17)
- Respiratory failure
- Restrictive lung disease (obesity, pulmonary fibrosis)

Cardiovascular
- Cardiac arrest
- Myocardial ischemia and/or infarction (see Chapter 28)

Neurologic
- Central nervous system dysfunction

Endocrine
- Carcinoid syndrome
- Pheochromocytoma
- Thyrotoxicosis

Musculoskeletal
- Malignant hyperthermia (see Chapter 27)
- Neuromuscular disease
- Shivering

Differential Diagnosis (continued)

Pharmacologic
- Neuroleptic malignant syndrome
- Residual anesthetic medications (eg, respiratory depressants, neuromuscular blocking drugs)

Other Considerations
- Anesthesia machine malfunction (eg, circuit problem, mechanical valve dysfunction, carbon dioxide absorbent exhausted, see Chapter 6)

- Esophageal intubation
- Hyperthermia (see Chapter 21)
- Infection and/or sepsis
- Massive hemorrhage (see Chapter 18)
- Reperfusion of ischemic tissue (removal of aortic cross-clamp, deflation of thigh cuff)
- Salicylate toxicity
- Systemic absorption of carbon dioxide during laparoscopic surgery

Suggested Readings

Bozimowski G. Clinical monitoring II: respiratory and metabolic systems. In: Nagelhout JJ, Plaus KL, eds. *Nurse Anesthesia.* 4th ed. St Louis, MO: Saunders Elsevier; 2010:337-347.

Greenberg SB, Murphy GS, Vender JS. Standard monitoring techniques. In: Barash PG, Cullen BF, Stoelting RK, Cahalan MK, Stock MC, eds. *Clinical Anesthesia.* 6th ed. Philadelphia, PA: Lippincott Williams & Wilkins; 2009:697-714.

Guyenet PG, Stornetta RL, Bayliss DA. Central respiratory chemoreception. *J Comp Neurol.* 2010;518(19):3883-3906.

Chapter 20
Hypertension

Treatment

- Assess blood pressure by noninvasive methods (ie, recheck measurement).
- Assess blood pressure by invasive methods (ie, assess level of transducer).
- Assess and treat potential causes of severe hypertension.
- Increase anesthetic depth.
- Provide adequate analgesia.
- Administer antihypertensive medications (drug and dose are dependent on the degree of hypertension and the patient's condition).
    - Vasodilators:
        - Nitroglycerin
        - Nitroprusside
        - Hydralazine
    - β-Blocking agents (eg, labetelol)
    - Calcium channel blocking agents (eg, nifedipine)
    - α-Blocking agents (eg, phenoxybenzamine)
    - Arterial line placement as needed

Physiology and Pathophysiology

Untreated and prolonged hypertension contributes to vascular pathology that can result in (1) atherosclerosis, (2) cerebral and aortic aneurysms, (3) myocardial hypertrophy, (4) myocardial ischemia and/or infarction, (5) hemorrhagic stroke, and (6) renal dysfunction and/or failure. The National Institutes of Health have created a classification system based on the degree of hypertension present (Table 20.1).

Arterial autoregulation is the ability of arteries to dilate and constrict over a range of blood pressures to maintain a constant blood flow. In humans, it is hypothesized that autoregulation occurs at MAPs of 60 to 150 mm Hg for cerebral arteries and 60 to 140 mm Hg for coronary arteries. Exceeding the maximal MAP in both the brain and the heart can lead to atherosclerosis and hemorrhagic stroke or myocardial ischemia. Increases in blood pressure (afterload) lead to increases in myocardial workload and oxygen demand. Severe hypertension can result in decreased stroke volume, cardiac output, and ultimately, myocardial performance.

Table 20.1. Classification of Blood Pressure for Adults Age 18 and Older

Category	Systolic blood pressure (mm Hg)		Diastolic blood pressure (mm Hg)
Normal	< 120	and	< 80
Prehypertension	120-139	or	80-89
Hypertension stage 1	140-159	or	90-99
Hypertension stage 2	≥ 160	or	≥ 100
Hypertension stage 3 (hypertensive crises)	> 180	or	> 110

Adapted from National Institutes of Health, National High Blood Pressure Program, JNC VII, 2003.

Signs and Symptoms

Respiratory
- Shortness of breath
- Tachypnea

Cardiovascular
- Bounding peripheral pulses
- Chest pain
- CHF
- Dysrhythmias
- Increased pulse pressure
- Increased systolic and/or diastolic blood pressure
- Myocardial ischemia and/or infarction
- Peripheral edema

Neurologic
- Altered level of consciousness
- Anxiety
- Blurred vision
- Headache
- Hemorrhagic stroke
- Papilledema

Renal
- Altered renal function
- Proteinuria

Other Considerations
- Epistaxis

Differential Diagnosis

Respiratory
- Airway obstruction (see Chapter 4)
- Hypercarbia (see Chapter 19)
- Hypoxia (see Chapter 24)
- Pulmonary edema

Cardiovascular
- Fluid overload
- Primary (essential) hypertension
- Renovascular hypertension

- Surgical compression of major vasculature (eg, aortic cross-clamp placement)
- SNS stimulation
  1. Surgical stimulation
  2. Inadequate depth of anesthesia
  3. Intubation
  4. Stimulation of the carina
  5. Emergence

Differential Diagnosis (continued)

Neurologic
- Autonomic hyperreflexia
- Increased intracranial pressure (Cushing reflex)

Endocrine
- Cushing syndrome
- Pheochromocytoma
- Thyrotoxicosis

Pharmacologic
- Adrenergic agonists (eg, ketamine)
- Drug withdrawal
- Medication error
- Naloxone
- Omission of prescribed anti-hypertensive medications
- Sympathomimetic drug abuse (eg, cocaine, methamphetamine)
- Vasopressor medications

Other Considerations
- Anxiety
- Distended bladder
- Equipment problem
  1. Arterial-line transducer inappropriately leveled (ie, below the level of the heart)
  2. Inadequately sized blood pressure cuff (ie, too small)
  3. Pressure on the blood pressure cuff by the surgical staff
- Hypoglycemia
- Malignant hyperthermia (see Chapter 27)
- Pain
- Preeclampsia or eclampsia (see Chapter 32)

Suggested Readings

Chobanian A, Bakris GL, Black HR, et al. The Seventh Report of the Joint National Committee on Prevention, Detection, Evaluation, and Treatment of High Blood Pressure. *Hypertension.* 2003;42(6): 1206-1252.

Elisha S. Cardiovascular anatomy, physiology, pathophysiology, and anesthesia management. In: Nagelhout JJ, Plaus KL, eds. *Nurse Anesthesia.* 4th ed. St Louis, MO: Saunders Elsevier; 2010:465-503.

Johnson B, Adi A, Licina MG, et al. Cardiac physiology. In: Kaplan JA, Reich DL, Lake CL, Konstadt SN, eds. *Kaplan's Cardiac Anesthesia.* 5th ed. Philadelphia, PA: Saunders Elsevier; 2006:71-89.

Chapter 21
Hyperthermia

Treatment

- Diagnose and treat underlying pathological state.
- Manage cardiac, pulmonary, and neurologic manifestations.
- Provide 100% oxygen.
- Use passive cooling methods:
    - Removal of clothing (surgical gown and blankets)
    - Removal of surgical drapes when possible
    - Decrease in OR temperature
- Use active cooling methods:
    - Forced-air cooling
    - Apply ice packs to head, armpits, and groin
    - Gastric lavage with cold, sterile water
    - Intravenous infusion of cold fluids
    - Irrigation of peritoneum with cold, sterile fluids when possible
- Monitor fluid and electrolyte status, and evaluate urine output and laboratory results.
- Monitor acid-base status by evaluating ABG results.
- Administer antipyretic medications (eg, acetaminophen, aspirin, NSAIDs).
- Administer antibiotic medication(s) when appropriate.

Physiology and Pathophysiology

Temperature regulation is maintained by the hypothalamus within a narrow range ($37°C \pm 0.5°C$). The hypothalamus (1) receives sensory input from central and peripheral thermoreceptors, (2) promotes conscious thermoregulatory behavior, and (3) initiates autonomic responses of thermoregulation based on the core body temperature. These autonomic responses include vasodilation and sweating.

Perioperative hyperthermia is defined as a core body temperature of greater than $38°C$. Factors that alter core body temperature include (1) basal metabolic rate and heat production, (2) perfusion to central and peripheral tissues, (3) hypothalamic temperature regulation, and (4) initiation of immune and inflammatory mechanisms that can cause hyperthermia. By increasing the body's metabolic rate, hyperthermia increases oxygen consumption and carbon dioxide production.

Signs and Symptoms

Respiratory
- Hypercarbia
- Tachypnea

Cardiovascular
- Diaphoresis
- Dysrhythmias
- Myocardial ischemia and/or infarction
- Tachycardia
- Vasodilation

Neurologic
- Altered level of consciousness
- Dizziness
- Febrile seizures
- Headache
- Syncope

Gastrointestinal
- Nausea and/or vomiting

Other Considerations
- Core body temperature higher than $38°C$
- Decreased urine output
- Increased perspiration
- Flushed, hot, and dry skin

Differential Diagnosis

Neurologic
- Altered hypothalamic function
  1. Encephalitis and meningitis
  2. Extremes of age
  3. Intracranial neoplasm
  4. Neurovascular pathology
  5. Traumatic brain injury
- Neuroleptic malignant syndrome

Endocrine
- Carcinoid syndrome
- Pheochromocytoma
- Thyrotoxicosis

Musculoskeletal
- Malignant hyperthermia (see Chapter 27)

Pharmacologic
- Acute drug intoxication (eg, cocaine and amphetamines)
- Cholinergic crisis
- Psychotropic medications

Other Considerations
- Immune and inflammatory mechanisms
  1. Early-stage sepsis
  2. Infection
  3. Transfusion reaction
- Inaccurate monitoring (eg, noncalibrated temperature probe)
- Prolonged environmental exposure to heat (eg, forced-air warming)
- Vascular hyperperfusion at site of monitoring

Suggested Readings

Bozimowski G. Clinical monitoring II: respiratory and metabolic systems. In: Nagelhout JJ, Plaus KL, eds. *Nurse Anesthesia.* 4th ed. St Louis, MO: Saunders Elsevier; 2010:337-347.

Larach MG, Brandom BW, Allen GC, Gronert GA, Lehman EB. Cardiac arrests and deaths associated with malignant hyperthermia in North America from 1987 to 2006: a report from The North American Malignant Hyperthermia Registry of the Malignant Hyperthermia Association of the United States. *Anesthesiology.* 2008;180(4): 603-611.

Merritt DR. Malignant hyperthermia: dantrolene. In: Ouellette RG, Joyce JA, eds. *Pharmacology for Nurse Anesthesiology.* Sudbury, MA: Jones & Bartlett; 2011:405-415.

Chapter 22
Hypotension

- Assess blood pressure by noninvasive methods (recheck measurement).
- Assess blood pressure by invasive methods (assess level of transducer).
- Increase F_{IO_2} to keep oxygen saturation > 90%.
- Assess peripheral pulses for severe hypotension.
- Call for help.
- Decrease or discontinue administration of anesthetic agents.
- Identify and treat the cause of severe hypotension.
- Expand intravascular volume:
  - Crystalloids
  - Colloids
  - Packed red blood cells if anemia is present
- Administer vasopressor(s) (drug and dose are dependent on the degree of hypotension and the patient's condition):
  - Ephedrine
  - Phenylephrine
  - Epinephrine
  - Vasopressin
- Insert arterial line.
- Insert second IV line or central line.
- Elevate lower extremities, use Trendelenburg position.
- Minimize PIP and decrease PEEP.
- Have rapid infusor available.
- Obtain laboratory analysis as needed (eg, hemoglobin and hematocrit, blood chemistry).
- Obtain diagnostic tests as needed (eg, ECG).
- Communicate with surgeon.

Physiology and Pathophysiology

Presently, a universally accepted definition for hypotension does not exist. Several guidelines have been suggested in an attempt to quantify intraoperative hypotension: (1) systolic blood pressure less than 80 to 90 mm Hg, (2) diastolic blood pressure less than 50 to 60 mm Hg, (3) MAP less than 50 to 60 mm Hg, and (4) greater than a 20% decrease in blood pressure as compared with preoperative values.

The greatest concern associated with severe hypotension includes cerebral and/or myocardial ischemia. Arterial autoregulation is the ability of arteries to dilate and constrict throughout a range of blood pressures to maintain constant blood flow to tissues. Cerebral and coronary artery autoregulation are hypothesized to occur in humans at MAP values of 60 to 150 mm Hg and 60 to 140 mm Hg, respectively. However, patients with cerebral and/or coronary artery pathology (ie, plaque lesions) may require a higher MAP to maintain adequate perfusion to vital organs.

Signs and Symptoms

Respiratory
- Airway obstruction (late sign, see Chapter 4)
- Shortness of breath
- Tachypnea

Cardiovascular
- Cardiac arrest
- Decreased capillary refill
- Decreased peripheral and/or central pulses
- Decreased systolic and/or diastolic blood pressure
- Dysrhythmias
- Low and/or narrowed pulse pressure
- Myocardial ischemia and/or infarction
- Pale skin/conjunctiva
- Poor capillary refill
- Tachycardia

Neurologic
- Altered level of consciousness (if conscious)
- Cerebral ischemia
- Ischemic stroke

Signs and Symptoms (continued)

Neurologic
- Nausea and/or vomiting (if conscious)

Renal
- Metabolic acidosis
- Oliguria

Differential Diagnosis

Respiratory
- Apnea
- Hypoxia (late sign)
- Use of PEEP
- Tension pneumothorax

Cardiovascular
- Acute heart valve insufficiency
- All shock states (see Chapter 34)
- Cardiac dysrhythmias (see Chapter 9)
- Cardiac tamponade (see Chapter 10)
- Cardiomyopathy
- CHF
- Embolism (see Chapter 17)
- Excessive abdominal pressure caused by pneumoperitoneum during laparoscopic surgery
- Hypovolemia
- Myocardial ischemia and/or infarction (see Chapter 28)

- Parasympathetic nervous system predominance (eg, vagal stimulation)
- Pressure by surgeon on major vascular structures
- Reflex bradycardia and/or vasodilation (eg, celiac reflex)
- Reperfusion of ischemic tissue (ie, removal of aortic cross-clamp)
- Valvular heart disease (eg, aortic, mitral, tricuspid, pulmonic)

Endocrine
- Acute adrenal crises (see Chapter 1)
- Adrenalectomy for pheo-chromocytoma (most likely to occur during period immediately following venous ligation)
- Hypothyroidism

Differential Diagnosis (continued)

Hematologic
- Anemia
- Hemorrhage
  (see Chapter 18)

Pharmacologic
- Anesthetic induction agents
- Benzodiazepines
- Excessive β blockade or
  calcium channel blockade
- Histamine release
  (eg, atracurium)
- Inhalation agents
- Local anesthetics (eg, spinal
  or epidural administration)
- Local anesthetic toxicity
  (see Chapter 26)
- Medication error
- Narcotics
- Reversal of heparin
  (eg, protamine)
- Total spinal anesthetic
  (see Chapter 36)
- Vasodilating agents
  (eg, nitroprusside)

Other Considerations
- Anaphylaxis (see Chapter 5)
- Assessment error (eg, blood
  pressure cuff too large,
  Arterial-line transducer
  above level of heart)
- Bone cement (polymethyl
  methacrylate)
- Hypermagnesemia
- Hypocalcemia
  (see Chapter 16)
- Hypoglycemia (rapid onset
  in neonates)
- Mechanical/surgical manipu-
  lation (eg, retractors)
- Pregnancy (eg, aortocaval
  compression)

Suggested Readings

Bijker JB, van Klei WA, Kappen TH, van Wolfswinkel L, Moons KG, Kalkman CJ. Incidence of intraoperative hypotension as a function of the chosen definition: literature definitions applied to a retrospective cohort using automated data collection. *Anesthesiology*. 2007;107(2):213-220.

Elisha S. Posterior spinal reconstructive surgery. In: Elisha S, ed. *Case Studies in Nurse Anesthesia*. Sudbury, MA: Jones & Bartlett; 2011:531-542.

Elisha S. Cardiovascular anatomy, physiology, pathophysiology, and anesthesia management. In: Nagelhout JJ, Plaus KL, eds. *Nurse Anesthesia*. 4th ed. St Louis, MO: Saunders Elsevier; 2010:465-503.

Chapter 23
Hypothermia

Treatment

- Treat underlying pathological state.
- Provide 100% oxygen.
- Use passive rewarming methods:
  - Increase ambient room temperature.
  - Cover the patient with warm clothing and/or blankets.
  - Cover the patient's head.
- Use active rewarming methods:
  - Forced-air warming
  - IV fluid warming
  - Warmed irrigation fluids
- Decrease distributive heat loss: forced-air warming a half-hour before induction.
- Decrease radiant heat loss:
  - Increase ambient room temperature.
  - Use radiant heat warmer.
  - Cover exposed areas when possible (especially the head).
- Decrease evaporative heat loss:
  - Minimize exposure of surgical site or exposed viscera.
  - Use semiclosed breathing circuit and low fresh gas flow.
  - Warm and humidify inspired gases.
- Decrease convection heat loss by covering patient.
- Decrease conductive heat loss:
  - Use warm irrigation fluids, IV fluids, and blood products.
  - Minimize direct contact with cold surfaces.
  - Monitor temperature in PACU.

Physiology and Pathophysiology

Temperature regulation of the human body to 37°C (98.6°F) is maintained by the hypothalamus. The hypothalamus (1) receives sensory input from central and peripheral thermoreceptors, (2) promotes conscious thermoregulatory behavior, and (3) initiates autonomic responses of thermoregulation based on the core body temperature. Autonomic responses to hypothermia include vasoconstriction, non-shivering thermogenesis, and shivering thermogenesis.

Perioperative hypothermia is defined as a core body temperature lower than 36°C. Conditions such as (1) decreased basal metabolic rate and heat production, (2) decreased perfusion to central and peripheral tissues, and (3) altered hypothalamic temperature regulation can predispose patients to hypothermic states. More commonly, perioperative hypothermia occurs as a result of 2 intraoperative phases: redistribution heat loss and continuous heat loss. Redistribution heat loss occurs after the induction of general or neuraxial anesthesia. It is caused by peripheral vasodilation and the transfer of heat from core to peripheral tissues. This transfer of heat results in a decrease in the core temperature by 1°C to 1.6°C. Mechanisms that promote continuous heat loss include the following:

- **Conduction:** Molecules at the surface of the skin or other exposed surfaces are transmitted to molecules of the medium adjacent to the skin.
- **Convection:** Heat is lost from movement of cold air over a warm surface.
- **Evaporation:** The vapor temperature of the body surface is different from that of the environment.
- **Radiation:** All objects that have a temperature above absolute zero produce electromagnetic radiation. Therefore, if the temperature of an object is lower than the temperature of the body, there is a net loss of heat from the body to the object (or the environment).

Signs and Symptoms

Respiratory
- Hypoxemia
- Ventilation and/or perfusion mismatch

Cardiovascular
- Cardiac dysfunction
- Dysrhythmias
- Myocardial infarction
- Peripheral vasoconstriction and/or piloerection

Neurologic
- Altered level of consciousness

Hematologic
- Decreased blood coagulation

Musculoskeletal
- Shivering

Pharmacologic
- Prolonged drug metabolism

Other Considerations
- Core body temperature lower than 36°C
- Skin cold to touch

Differential Diagnosis

Cardiovascular
- Shock states (see Chapter 34)

Neurologic
- Depressed hypothalamic function
  1. Anesthetic medications
  2. Extremes of age
  3. Intracranial neoplasm
  4. Neurovascular pathology
  5. Traumatic brain injury

Endocrine
- Myxedema coma
- Panhypopituitarism

Other Considerations
- Continuous heat loss
  1. Conduction: Rapid infusion of cold IV fluids and blood products and/or exposure to cold OR equipment such as OR table
  2. Convection: Prolonged exposure to circulating cool air
  3. Evaporation: Cold and un-humidified inspired gases and/or exposed viscera

Differential Diagnosis (continued)

Other Considerations

   4. Radiation: Surgery of prolonged duration or increased complexity
   • Exposure to extreme cold temperatures
   • Inaccurate monitoring (ie, noncalibrated temperature probe)

• Permissive hypothermia
   1. Cardiopulmonary bypass
   2. Deep hypothermic circulatory arrest
   3. Neurosurgical hypothermic techniques
• Redistribution heat loss from inadequate forced-air warming a half-hour before induction
• Vascular insufficiency at monitoring site

Suggested Readings

Bozimowski G. Clinical monitoring II: respiratory and metabolic systems. In: Nagelhout JJ, Plaus KL, eds. *Nurse Anesthesia.* 4th ed. St Louis, MO: Saunders Elsevier; 2010:337-347.

Insler SR, Sessler DI. Perioperative thermoregulation and temperature monitoring. *Anesthesiol Clin.* 2006;24(4):823-837.

Welch TC. A common sense approach to hypothermia. *AANA J.* 2002;70(3):227-231.

Chapter 24
Hypoxia

Treatment

- Ventilate with 100% oxygen.
- Determine and treat the specific cause of hypoxia.
- Manually ventilate, listen to breath sounds, and confirm $ETCO_2$.
- Intubate and confirm correct placement of ETT.
- Verify pulse oximetry reading.
- Check anesthesia breathing circuit (ie, disconnect, kinks, holes).
- Obtain ABG.
- Administer bronchodilators as needed.
- Consider CPAP if the patient is not intubated.
- Consider PEEP if patient is intubated.
- Perform cardiac resuscitation per American Heart Association ACLS or PALS protocol as necessary.
- Obtain chest radiograph.
- Obtain ECG.

Miscellaneous Treatments
- Consider tracheal suctioning, bronchial lavage, corticosteroids, and/or antibiotics for gastric aspiration.
- Descend to lower altitude for high-altitude hypoxia.
- Administer hyperbaric oxygen therapy for carbon dioxide or cyanide poisoning.
- Consider hydroxocobalamin or sodium thiosulfate for cyanide poisoning.
- Bronchoscopy
- Needle decompression and chest tube placement, if evidence of pneumothorax exists.

Physiology and Pathophysiology

Hypoxia is defined as a low blood oxygen content and is assessed by an Spo_2 less than 90% or Pao_2 less than 60 mm Hg. Oxygen is a vital component necessary for cellular metabolism and ATP production. When oxygen concentrations are decreased, anaerobic metabolism ensues, resulting in cellular dysfunction, acidosis, multiorgan failure, and eventually death. Hypoxia is divided into 4 categories, which include (1) anemic hypoxia, (2) hypoxic hypoxia, (3) stagnant hypoxia, and (4) histotoxic hypoxia. Possible causes of hypoxia are included in Table 24.1.

Anemic hypoxia refers to any condition that affects the production or function of the red blood cell and hemoglobin molecules. *Hypoxic hypoxia* includes conditions that decrease the amount of oxygen reaching the lungs and subsequently diffusing into the blood. *Stagnant hypoxia* is any disorder that leads to inadequate tissue oxygenation from a reduction in blood flow. Finally, *histotoxic hypoxia* causes impaired oxygen use at the cellular level, specifically the inhibition of cytochrome oxidase.

In the pediatric population, the SNS is functionally immature, resulting in parasympathetic nervous system predominance; the ensuing initial physical signs associated with hypoxia may include respiratory arrest, bradycardia, and cardiac arrest.

Table 24.1. Types and Causes of Hypoxia

Anemic hypoxia
> Carbon monoxide poisoning
> Chemotherapy
> Hemorrhage
> Renal disease
> Sickle cell disease
> Thalassemia

Hypoxic hypoxia
> Alterations in nerve transmission (eg, neurogenic shock, recurrent laryngeal nerve injury, phrenic nerve dysfunction, local anesthetic induced nerve blockade)
> CNS depression (eg, medications, trauma, hypoperfusion)
> Decreased F_{IO_2} (eg, absence of ventilation, hypoxic mixture, high altitude)
> Decreased functional residual capacity (eg, obesity, pregnancy, restrictive lung disease)
> Equipment malfunction (eg, circuit leak or disconnection, kink in ETT, pipeline failure)
> Hypoventilation
> Obstructive lung disease (eg, COPD, asthma)
> Respiratory muscle incompetence or failure (eg, diaphragmatic trauma, high spinal anesthetic)
> Thoracic structural malformations (eg, scoliosis, thoracic trauma)

Upper airway conditions:
> Foreign body
> Laryngospasm
> Mass and/or thyroid goiter
> Obstructive sleep apnea
> Upper respiratory tract infection

Lower airway conditions:
> Inflammation (eg, ARDS, cystic fibrosis)
> Pneumothorax, hemothorax or tension pneumothorax
> Pneumonia
> Pulmonary contusion
> Restrictive and/or obstructive lung disease

Increased dead space ventilation:
> Pulmonary embolism
> Pulmonary vasoconstriction

Increased intrapulmonary shunt:
> Aspiration with direct bronchiolar and alveolar tissue damage
> Atelectasis
> Bronchospasm
> Pulmonary edema

Abbreviations: CNS, central nervous system; F_{IO_2} fraction of inspired oxygen; COPD, chronic obstructive pulmonary disease; ETT, endotracheal tube; ARDS, acute respiratory distress syndrome; CHF, congestive heart failure.

Table 24.1. Types and Causes of Hypoxia (continued)

Stagnant hypoxia
- Embolism
- Polycythemia
- Pump failure (eg, CHF, myocardial infarction, trauma, cardiac tamponade)
- Severe hypotension (eg, hemorrhage, sepsis, anaphylaxis, neurogenic shock)

Histotoxic hypoxia
- Alcohol poisoning
- Carbon monoxide poisoning
- Cyanide poisoning
- Hydrogen sulfide poisoning

Abbreviations: CNS, central nervous system; FIO_2 fraction of inspired oxygen; COPD, chronic obstructive pulmonary disease; ETT, endotracheal tube; ARDS, acute respiratory distress syndrome; CHF, congestive heart failure.

Signs and Symptoms

- Early signs:
  1. Tachypnea
  2. Tachycardia
  3. Hypertension
- Late signs:
  1. Bradypnea and/or apnea
  2. Bradycardia
  3. Hypotension

Respiratory
- Cyanosis
- Decreased, abnormal, or absent breath sounds
- Decreased arterial oxygen pressure (PaO_2 < 60 mm Hg)
- Decreased pulse oximetry reading (SpO_2 < 90%)
- Elevated methemoglobin and/or carboxyhemoglobin levels

Cardiovascular
- Dysrhythmia
- Hypoventilation
- Increased, decreased, or absent $ETCO_2$
- Pallor

Neurologic
- Agitation
- Headache
- Nausea and/or vomiting
- Seizures
- Somnolence leading to unconsciousness

Musculoskeletal
- Visual assessment of altered anatomy of the airway or chest

Differential Diagnosis

Respiratory
- Airway fire (see Chapter 3)
- Airway obstruction (see Chapter 4)
- Aspiration (see Chapter 2)
- Atelectasis
- Bronchospasm (see Chapter 8)
- Decreased F_{IO_2} administration (eg, hypoxic mixture, high altitude)
- Decreased functional residual capacity (eg, obesity, pregnancy)
- Esophageal and/or endobronchial intubation
- Hypoventilation (residual anesthetic effects, inadequate ventilation settings)
- Hypoxic pulmonary vasoconstriction inhibition
- Interstitial lung disease
- Intrapulmonary shunt
- Obstructive lung disease (eg, asthma, COPD)
- Pneumonia
- Pneumothorax (see Chapter 31)
- Pulmonary edema
- Pulmonary embolism (see Chapter 17)
- Smoke inhalation
- Traumatic lung injury

Cardiovascular
- Cardiac tamponade
- Congestive heart failure
- Intracardiac shunt
- Myocardial ischemia and/or infarction (see Chapter 28)

Neurologic
- Cerebral herniation
- Neuromuscular disorder (eg, myasthenia gravis, Parkinson disease exacerbation, multiple sclerosis, Guillain-Barré syndrome)

Endocrine
- Acute pancreatitis
- Pheochromocytoma
- Thyrotoxicosis

Hematologic
- Transfusion reaction from blood product administration

Musculoskeletal
- External airway compression (tumor)
- Hypermetabolic states (malignant hyperthermia)
- Structural abnormalities (eg, scoliosis, thoracic cage malformations)
- Trauma (eg, diaphragmatic rupture, rib fracture, sternal fracture)

Differential Diagnosis (continued)

Pharmacologic
- Alcohol intoxication
- CNS depressants (eg, opioids, benzodiazepines, barbiturates, marijuana)
- Cyanide poisoning (eg, sodium nitroprusside infusions, smoke inhalation, chemicals in the workplace)
- Local anesthetic toxicity (see Chapter 26)
- Methylene blue or indigo carmine

Other Considerations
- All shock states (see Chapter 34)
- Anaphylaxis (see Chapter 5)
- Anesthesia machine failure (see Chapter 6)
- Carbon monoxide poisoning
- Equipment malfunction (eg, pulse oximetry, mass spectrometry, anesthesia machine dysfunction, see Chapter 6)
- Sepsis
- Type of surgical procedure (eg, pneumonectomy, thoracic surgery, cardiac surgery)

Suggested Readings

Blum JM, Blank R, Rochlen LR. Anesthesia for patients requiring advanced ventilatory support. *Anesthesiol Clin.* 2010;28(1):25-38.

Hamel J. A review of acute cyanide poisoning with a treatment update. *Crit Care Nurse.* 2011;31(1):72-82.

Odom-Forren J. Postanesthesia recovery. In: Nagelhout JJ, Plaus KL, eds. *Nurse Anesthesia.* 4th ed. St Louis, MO: Saunders Elsevier; 2010:1218-1238.

Chapter 25
Laryngospasm

Treatment

- Provide F_{IO_2} at 100%.
- Confirm oropharyngeal patency (eg, oral airway).
- Jaw thrust with pressure posterior to mandibular angle (eg, "laryngospasm notch")
- Manual ventilation with continuous positive airway pressure
- For persistent, inadequate ventilation and/or oxygenation:
  1. Administer succinylcholine.
     — Adult dose, 0.2 to 0.5 mg/kg, IV
     — Pediatric dose, 4 to 5 mg/kg IM, 2 to 3 mg/kg IV (Concomitant administration of atropine is necessary in pediatric patients to avoid bradycardia.)
  2. If succinylcholine is contraindicated, administer rocuronium (1.0 - 1.2 mg/kg, IV).
  3. Monitor for negative-pressure pulmonary edema.

Physiology and Pathophysiology

Laryngospasm is a primitive, protective laryngeal reflex that occurs in response to a variety of noxious stimuli (eg, water, mucus, and blood). The exact neural pathway and mechanical mechanism by which laryngospasm occurs is not definitively understood. Laryngospasm is most probably caused by the combined contraction of multiple laryngeal muscles. One possibility for this physiological reflex is that noxious stimuli transmit an afferent sensory response from

Physiology and Pathophysiology (continued)

the glottis to the internal branch of the superior laryngeal nerve, and an efferent motor response via the external branch of the superior laryngeal nerve activates the cricothyroid muscles, stimulating them to contract, resulting in laryngospasm.

Signs and Symptoms

Respiratory
- Abnormal or absent $ETCO_2$ waveform
- Cyanosis
- Desaturation
- Hypercarbia
- Hypoxemia
- Inadequate chest rise
- Inadequate face mask ventilation
- Inspiratory or expiratory stridor (ie, partial laryngospasm)
- Intercostal and/or suprasternal inspiratory retractions
- Negative-pressure pulmonary edema
  1. Bilateral rales
  2. Radiographic evidence of pulmonary edema
  3. Pink frothy or exudative pulmonary secretions
- Oral secretions/blood
- Paradoxical movements of chest and abdomen

Cardiovascular
- Bradycardia (late sign of hypoxia)
- Increased blood pressure
- Tachycardia (early sign of hypoxia)

Differential Diagnosis

Respiratory
- Abnormal airway anatomy
  1. Mediastinal mass
  2. Malignancy
  3. Airway trauma
- Bronchospasm
  (see Chapter 8)
- Foreign body (eg, retained throat pack)
- Neck hematoma
- Pneumothorax
- Subcutaneous emphysema
- Supraglottic and or subglottic edema
- Upper airway obstruction
  (see Chapter 4)

Other Considerations
- Anaphylactic reaction
  (see Chapter 5)
- Hypocalcemia
- Insertion of oral and/or nasal airway
- Light anesthesia

Suggested Readings

Al-alami AA, Zestos MM, Baraka AS. Pediatric laryngospasm: prevention and treatment. *Curr Opin Anaesthesiol.* 2009;22(3):388-395.

Davis PJ, Lerman J, Tofovic SP, Cook DR. Pharmacology of pediatric anesthesia. In: Motoyama EK, Davis PJ, eds. *Smith's Anesthesia for Infants and Children.* 7th ed. Philadelphia, PA: Mosby Elsevier; 2006:177-238.

Sharma A. Cleft palate. In: Yao FSF, ed. *Yao & Artusio's Anesthesiology: Problem-Oriented Patient Management.* 6th ed. Philadelphia, PA: Lippincott Williams & Wilkins; 2008:1049-1060.

Welliver MD, Welliver DC. Vocal cord polyp removal with laser. In: Elisha S, ed. *Case Studies in Nurse Anesthesia.* Sudbury, MA: Jones & Bartlett; 2011:41-50.

Chapter 26
Local Anesthetic Toxicity

Treatment

If *mild to moderate* signs and symptoms of LA toxicity occur:
• Stop LA injection.

• Administer 100% oxygen.

• Assess airway, breathing, and circulation.

• Administer anticonvulsant drugs to increase seizure threshold (a single drug or a combination).

   1. benzodiazepine

   2. propofol

If *severe* LA toxicity occurs and/or patient condition deteriorates:
• Call for help.

• Stop LA injection.

• Monitor airway and/or breathing.

   1. Intubate the trachea.

   2. Ventilate to prevent hypoxia, acidosis, and ion trapping.

• Assess circulation.

   1. Administer IV fluid bolus.

   2. Administer anticonvulsant medications as above.

   3. For persistent tonic-clonic seizure activity, consider neuromuscular blockade.

   4. For hypotension, administer vasopressors and/or inotropic medications.

   5. For severe and/or sustained bradycardia, administer atropine.

Treatment (continued)

6. For cardiac arrest caused by LA toxicity:
   — Perform cardiac resuscitation per American Heart Association protocol.
   — Administer Intralipids:
     i. Intralipid 20% IV bolus (1.5 mL/kg for 1 minute)
     ii. Intralipid 20% IV infusion (0.25 mL/kg/minute)
     iii. Repeat Intralipid 20% IV bolus every 3 to 5 minutes (1.5-3.0 mL/kg)
     iv. Maximum Intralipid dose, 8 mL/kg

Physiology and Pathophysiology

Local anesthetic medications attenuate action potential propagation along nerves by inhibiting depolarization. Thus, motor, sensory, and vascular sympathetic tone is inhibited. The brain, compared with the heart, is more sensitive to the effects of elevated plasma concentrations of LA. This explains why neurologic signs and symptoms increase and progress as the LA plasma concentration of the LA increases until finally, cardiotoxicity ensues. Hypoxia, hypercarbia, and acidosis potentiate cardiotoxicity. Suspected causes of cardiotoxicity include LA blockade of cardiac sodium, potassium, and calcium channels and cardiomyocyte mitochondrial inhibition. Because of its high potency, bupivacaine has been most often implicated in cases of cardiac arrest caused by LA toxicity. LA toxicity is dependent on multiple factors, including the following:

- The specific LA medication (LA with greater potency, such as bupivacaine, will cause toxicity at lower plasma concentrations)
- The speed of absorption of LA into plasma

Physiology and Pathophysiology (continued)

- Total LA plasma concentration (mg/kg dose)
- Addition of epinephrine to LA
- A person's ability to metabolize and excrete the LA

To prevent LA toxicity:

- Aspirate before LA injection to check for blood and/or CSF.
- For epidural or regional anesthesia, inject LA in 3- to 5-mL increments.
- Add epinephrine into LA solutions for injection to assess for increased heart rate during epidural dosing.
- Talk to the patient to assess level of consciousness and other signs and symptoms associated with neurologic LA toxicity.
- Calculate the toxic dose per patient's kilogram weight before LA administration or additional LA infiltration by the surgeon.

Recent reports concerning LA toxicity suggest the most common manifestations include immediate seizures and/or cardiac arrest.

Signs and Symptoms

Mild to moderate neurologic manifestations of LA toxicity:

- Circumoral and/or tongue numbness
- Disorientation
- Lightheadedness
- Metallic taste in mouth
- Muscular twitching
- Tinnitus
- Visual disturbances

Severe neurologic manifestations of LA toxicity:

- Coma
- Respiratory arrest
- Seizures
- Unconsciousness

Exceedingly high LA plasma concentrations affecting cardiac electrophysiology and/or contractility:

- Cardiac arrest
- Dysrhythmias
- Ventricular fibrillation
- Ventricular tachycardia

Differential Diagnosis

Respiratory
- Hyperventilation and/or panic disorder
- Hypoxia (see Chapter 24)

Cardiovascular
- Myocardial ischemia and/or infarction (see Chapter 28)
- Severe hypotension (see Chapter 22)

Neurologic
- Cerebrovascular accident in evolution
- Neurogenic shock (see Chapter 34)
- Preexisting neurologic disorders (eg, seizure disorder, intracranial mass)

Pharmacologic
- Local anesthetic overdose
- Regional anesthesia administration (eg, intravascular injection)
- Sympathomimetic drug use (eg, cocaine, methamphetamine)
- Total spinal and/or epidural blockade (see Chapter 36)
- Vasovagal reaction

Other Considerations
- Acidosis
- Anaphylaxis (see Chapter 5)
- Eclampsia (see Chapter 32)
- Hyponatremia (ie, TURP syndrome, see Chapter 38)

Suggested Readings

Candela D, Louart G, Bousquet PJ, et al. Reversal of bupivacaine-induced cardiac electrophysiologic changes by two lipid emulsions in anesthetized and mechanically ventilated piglets. *Anesth Analg.* 2010;110(5):1473-1479.

DiGregorio G, Neal JM, Rosenquist RW, Weinberg GL. Clinical presentation of local anesthetic systemic toxicity. *Reg Anesth Pain Med.* 2010;35(2):181-187.

Suggested Readings (continued)

McLeod GA, Butterworth JF, Wildsmith JAW. Local anesthetic systemic toxicity. In: Cousins MJ, Carr DB, Horlocker TT, Bridenbaugh PO, eds. *Cousins and Bridenbaugh's Neural Blockade In Clinical Anesthesia and Pain Medicine.* 4th ed. Philadelphia, PA: Lippincott Williams & Wilkins; 2009:114-132.

Nagelhout JJ. Local anesthetics. In: Nagelhout JJ, Plaus KL, eds. *Nurse Anesthesia.* 4th ed. St Louis, MO: Saunders Elsevier; 2010:142-164.

Neal JM, Bernards CM. Butterworth JF IV, et al. ASRA practice advisory on local anesthetic systemic toxicity. *Reg Anesth Pain Med.* 2010;35(2):152-161.

Chapter 27
Malignant Hyperthermia

Treatment

- Call for help.
- Communicate with surgeon.
- Discontinue inhalation agent administration.
- Discontinue succinylcholine administration.
- Ventilate using new anesthesia circuit with high-flow 100% oxygen.
- Increase minute ventilation.
- Administer dantrolene IV (2.5 mg/kg), increasing until symptoms associated with hypermetabolism improve (may exceed 10 mg/kg).
- Consider sodium bicarbonate, 1 to 2 mEq/kg, for acidosis.
- Administer cooling measures:
  - Forced-air cooling
  - Cooled IV fluids
  - Intraperitoneal lavage
  - Intragastric lavage
- Use invasive monitoring (arterial line, second large-bore IV line).
- Administer IV fluids and place urinary catheter to monitor urine output.
- Treat metabolic acidosis.
- Treat hyperkalemia, if present.
- Administer calcium chloride (10 mg/kg).
- Administer sodium bicarbonate (1-2 mEq/kg).
- Administer insulin (10 U regular) with 1 to 2 amp of $D_{50}W$.
- Treat dysrhythmias, if present.

Treatment (continued)

- Avoid use of calcium channel blockers.
- Obtain serial laboratory tests:
  o ABG
  o electrolytes (potassium)
  o coagulation panel
  o CK
  o serum/urine myglobin
- Transfer to ICU.
- Consult with Malignant Hyperthermia Association of the United States (MHAUS) 1-800-MHHYPER.
- Perform cardiac resuscitation per American Heart Association ACLS or PALS protocol as necessary.

Physiology and Pathophysiology

Malignant hyperthermia is an uncommon genetic disorder that is caused by sensitization of RYR receptor 1 that reside on the sarcoplasmic reticulum within skeletal muscle. The anesthetic triggering agents (inhalation agents and succinylcholine) interact with RYR receptor 1 to cause excessive release and inhibition of resequestration of calcium, which results in skeletal muscle tetany. The increased oxygen demand and need for ATP by skeletal muscles results in a hypermetabolic state that, if not reversed, leads to cellular hypoxia, acidosis, and death. The severity of the symptoms exhibited is proportional to the amount of intracellular calcium released. Pathological conditions that predispose patients to developing malignant hyperthermia include central core disease, multiple types of muscular dystrophy (Duchenne or Becker), King-Denborough syndrome, myopathic

Physiology and Pathophysiology (continued)

disease, and sarcoplasmic reticulum ATP deficiency. The onset and severity of the signs and symptoms are variable.

Signs and Symptoms

Respiratory
- Elevated ETCO$_2$ (most sensitive and specific sign)
- Decreased Pao$_2$
- Increased Paco$_2$

Cardiovascular
- Cardiac arrest
- Diaphoresis
- Dysrhythmias
- Hypertension
- Mottled and cyanotic skin
- Tachycardia

Musculoskeletal
- Elevated CK level
- Elevated urine and serum myoglobin levels
- Generalized muscle rigidity
- Masseter muscle spasm
- Myoglobinuria
- Rhabdomyolysis

Other Considerations
- Dark urine
- Decreased urine output
- Exhausted carbon dioxide absorbent
- Hyperkalemia
- Hyperthermia
- Metabolic acidosis

Differential Diagnosis

Respiratory
- Endobronchial intubation and/or tube migration
- Hypercarbia (see Chapter 19)
- Hypoventilation

Cardiovascular
- Shock states (see Chapter 34)

Neurologic
- Hypothalamic lesions

Renal
- Acute renal dysfunction (see Chapter 33)

Endocrine
- Carcinoid syndrome
- Pheochromocytoma
- Thyrotoxicosis

Pharmacologic
- Atropine (central anticholinergic syndrome)
- Drug error
- Monoamine oxidase inhibitors

- Psychotropic medications such as haloperidol, chlorpromazine, metoclopramide, lithium (neuroleptic malignant syndrome)
- Sympathomimetics
  1. Therapeutic medications (eg, epinephrine)
  2. Illegal drug use (eg, cocaine, methamphetamines)

Other Considerations
- Error with carbon dioxide sampling (see Chapter 6)
- Exhausted carbon dioxide absorbent (see Chapter 6)
- Hyperthermia (see Chapter 21)
- Inadequate anesthesia during surgical stimulation
- Systemic absorption of carbon dioxide during laparoscopic procedures

Suggested Readings

Karlet MC. Musculoskeletal system anatomy, physiology, pathophysiology, and anesthesia management. In: Nagelhout JJ, Plaus KL, eds. *Nurse Anesthesia.* 4th ed. St Louis, MO: Saunders Elsevier; 2010: 780-801.

Malignant Hyperthermia Association of the United States (MHAUS). http://www.mhaus.org/. Accessed April 17, 2011.

Rosenberg H, Brandom BW, Sambuughin N. Malignant hyperthermia and other inherited disorders. In: Barash PG, Cullen BF, Stoelting RK, Cahalan MK, Stock MC, eds. *Clinical Anesthesia.* 6th ed. Philadelphia, PA: Lippincott Williams & Wilkins; 2009:598-621.

Chapter 28
Myocardial Ischemia and Infarction

Treatment

- Inform the surgeon.
- Monitor and support airway, breathing, and circulation.
- Confirm diagnosis:
  - Assess for signs and symptoms (see Signs and Symptoms).
  - Obtain 12-lead ECG.
  - Perform transesophageal or transthoracic echocardiography.
  - Obtain cardiac enzymes level.
- Administer 100% FIO_2.
- Administer pharmacologic treatment (see Table 28.2).
- Consult with a cardiologist.
- Consider using invasive monitoring (ie, arterial line).
- Use American Heart Association management for acute coronary syndrome.
- Perform cardiac resuscitation per American Heart Association ACLS protocol as necessary.
- Prepare for higher level of cardiac care:
  - Cardiac catheterization
  - Fibrinolytic therapy
  - Antithrombotic therapy

Physiology and Pathophysiology

During anesthesia and surgery, physiological stress causes hemodynamic variability throughout the perioperative process. When factors are present that increase myocardial oxygen demand in relation to supply, ischemia, and infarction can occur. These factors that influence myocardial supply and demand are listed in Table 28.1. When myocardial oxygen deprivation occurs, myocardial excitation contractile coupling is inhibited because of a lack of ATP production. Myocardial wall motion abnormalities ensue, and if untreated, cardiogenic shock can occur. Rapid diagnosis and treatment are essential to inhibit myocardial damage and preserve myocardial function. Acute ECG changes, dysrhythmias, and hypotension are classic signs of cardiac ischemia or infarction. Treatment strategies for management are included in Table 28.2.

Table 28.1. Factors that Influence Myocardial Oxygen Supply and Demand

Supply	Demand
Decreased heart rate	Increased heart rate
Coronary blood flow	Preload
Diastolic blood pressure	Afterload
Oxygenated hemoglobin	Contractility

Table 28.2. Treatment for Intraoperative Myocardial Ischemia or Infarction

Hemodynamic event	Therapy	Pharmacologic action
Hypertension and tachycardia	Increase anesthetic depth.	Decreases SNS reactivity
	IV β-blockade	Decreases inotropy and/or chronotropy
	IV nitroglycerin	Decreases preload and/or wall tension, dilates epicardial vessels
Normotension and tachycardia	Adequate anesthetic depth?	Decreases SNS reactivity
	IV β-blockade	Decreases inotropy and/or chronotropy
Hypertension and normal heart rate	Increase anesthetic depth.	Decreases SVR, myocardial depression
	IV nitroglycerin or nicardipine	Decreases preload and/or wall tension, dilates epicardial vessels
Hypotension and tachycardia	IV fluid bolus	Increases intravascular volume
	Decrease anesthetic depth.	Increases SVR
	Phenylephrine	Increases SVR
	IV nitroglycerin when normotensive	Decreases preload and/or wall tension, dilates epicardial vessels
Hypotension and bradycardia	Ensure oxygenation.	Hypoxia of the cardioaccelerator center
	Decrease anesthetic depth.	Increases SVR
	IV ephedrine	Increases SVR, increases inotropy and/or chronotropy
	IV epinephrine	Increases inotropy and/or chronotropy
	IV atropine	Decreases PNS reactivity
	IV nitroglycerin when normotensive	Decreases preload and/or wall tension, dilates epicardial vessels

Abbreviations: SNS, sympathetic nervous system; SVR, systemic vascular resistance; PNS, parasympathetic nervous system.

Table 28.2. Treatment for Intraoperative Myocardial Ischemia or Infarction (continued)

Hemodynamic event	Therapy	Pharmacologic action
Hypotension and normal heart rate	Decrease anesthetic depth.	Increases SVR
	IV phenylephrine	Increases SVR
	IV ephedrine	Increases SVR, increases inotropy and/or chronotropy
	IV epinephrine	Increases SVR, increases inotropy and/or chronotropy
	IV nitroglycerin when normotensive	Decreases preload and/or wall tension, dilates epicardial vessels
Ischemia and/or infarction without hemodynamic abnormality	IV nitroglycerin	Decreases preload and/or wall tension, dilates epicardial vessels
	IV nicardipine	Decreases preload and/or wall tension, dilates epicardial vessels

Abbreviations: SNS, sympathetic nervous system; SVR, systemic vascular resistance; PNS, parasympathetic nervous system.

Signs and Symptoms

Respiratory
- Hypercarbia
- Hypoxia (see Chapter 24)
- Rales
- Respiratory arrest
- Shortness of breath
- Tachypnea

Cardiovascular
- Cardiac arrest
- Cardiogenic shock

- Chest pain with or without radiation
- Pain in jaw and/or left arm
- CHF
- Decreased capillary refill
- Decreased peripheral pulses
- Diaphoresis
- ECG
  1. Dysrhythmias
  2. ST segment elevation or depression

Signs and Symptoms (continued)

Cardiovascular

   3. New onset AV or bundle branch block

   4. New onset T-wave inversion

- Elevated cardiac troponin and CK-MB
- Hemodynamic profile
  1. Tachycardia or bradycardia
  2. Hypertension or hypotension
  3. Increased PCWP
  4. Increased CVP
  5. Increased systemic vascular resistance
- New onset cardiac murmur
- Ventricular wall motion abnormalities on transesophageal echocardiography

Neurologic

- Altered consciousness or loss of consciousness
- Dizziness
- Nausea and/or vomiting
- Syncope

Differential Diagnosis

Respiratory

- Pleuritis
- Pulmonary embolism (see Chapter 17)

Cardiovascular

- Acute aortic dissection
- Cardiac tamponade (see Chapter 10)
- Coronary artery vasospasm
- Costochondritis
- Pericarditis
- Shock states (see Chapter 34)

Neurologic

- Anxiety

Gastrointestinal

- Dyspepsia and/or gastroesophageal reflux disease

Other Considerations

- Acute adrenal crises (see Chapter 1)
- Anaphylaxis (see Chapter 5)
- Cholecystitis
- Intercostal muscle spasm
- Pancreatitis
- Trauma (eg, cardiac contusion)

Suggested Readings

Bhatt DL. Acute coronary syndrome update for hospitalists. *J Hosp Med.* 2010;5(suppl 4):S15-S21.

Elisha S. Cardiovascular anatomy, physiology, pathophysiology, and anesthesia management. In: Nagelhout JJ, Plaus KL, eds. *Nurse Anesthesia.* 4th ed. St Louis, MO: Saunders Elsevier; 2010:465-503.

Kampine JP, Stowe DF, Pagel PS. Cardiovascular anatomy and physiology. In: Barash PG, Cullen BF, Stoelting RK, Cahalan MK, Stock MC, eds. *Clinical Anesthesia.* 6th ed. Philadelphia, PA: Lippincott Williams & Wilkins; 2009:209-232.

London M, Mittnacht A, Kaplan JA. Anesthesia for myocardial revascularization. In: Kaplan JA, Reich DL, Lake CL, Konstadt SN, eds. *Kaplan's Cardiac Anesthesia.* 5th ed. Philadelphia, PA: Saunders Elsevier; 2006:585-643.

Chapter 29
Obstetric Hemorrhage

Treatment

Preoperative
- Identify risk factors for maternal hemorrhage (eg, uterine atony, abnormal placental attachment).
- Perform a thorough history and physical examination.
- Evaluate the patient for a potentially difficult airway.
- Consider administering pharmacologic prophylaxis for gastric aspiration.
- Maintain left uterine displacement until delivery of the fetus.
- Maintain effective communication with the surgical team.
- Avoid lethal triad:
  1. Acidosis
  2. Hypothermia
  3. Coagulopathy
- Refer to Chapter 18, Hemorrhage.
- Refer to Chapter 14, Disseminated Intravascular Coagulation.

Intraoperative
- Call for help.
- Remain cognizant of airway and breathing (possibility of difficult airway):
  1. Secure airway and provide adequate ventilation when there is potential or actual loss of consciousness, severe respiratory distress, and/or cardiovascular collapse.
  2. Perform a rapid-sequence induction with cricoid pressure.
  3. Consider ketamine or etomidate for induction.
  4. Provide FIO_2 at 100%.

Treatment (continued)

- Maintain adequate circulation:
  1. Provide volume replacement therapy (eg, crystalloids, colloids, blood, and/or blood products).
  2. Administer pharmacological support (eg, vasopressors, inotropic medications)
- Prevent hypothermia:
  - Use forced-air convective warmer.
  - Use fluid warmer.
- Administer blood, FFP, and platelets guided by hemoglobin values and hemodynamics.
- Provide pharmacologic and/or uterotonic treatment for uterine atony:
  1. Oxytocin: 10 to 40 U/L of normal saline or lactated Ringer's solution
  2. Methergine: 0.2 mg IM every 4 hours up to 1 mg total (caution if patient has hypertension)
  3. Hemabate: 0.25 mg IM or intrauterine every 20 to 30 minutes up to 2 mg total (caution if patient has asthma or hypertension)
  4. Cytotec: 1 mg total by rectum or sublingual
- Surgeon should consider surgical treatment for uterine hemorrhage:
  1. Manual pressure
  2. B-Lynch suture
  3. Intrauterine balloon tamponade
  4. Embolization of uterine or iliac arteries with balloon occlusion catheters
  5. Mechanical clamping of uterine or iliac arteries
  6. Emergency hysterectomy

Treatment (continued)

- Accurately assess blood loss:
  1. Suction canister
  2. Kidney basins
  3. Visual assessment of surgical field, surgical drapes, gowns, and OR floor
  4. Weighing of all surgical sponges and sanitary pads. Laparotomy sponge (18" × 18") and sanitary pads can each retain up to 100 mL when saturated.
- Obtain serial laboratory tests:
  - CBC count
  - PT/PTT/INR
  - Fibrinogen level
  - Electrolyte level
  - ABG measurement
- Perform cardiac resuscitation per American Heart Association ACLS protocol as necessary.

Physiology and Pathophysiology

Obstetric hemorrhage is a major cause of maternal morbidity and mortality and may occur during the antepartum, intrapartum, or postpartum period. Obstetric patients have an increased circulating blood volume and may exhibit signs and symptoms of hypovolemia (eg, tachycardia and hypotension) only when intravascular volume depletion is extreme. Therefore, it is imperative that an accurate assessment of blood loss be performed and immediate treatment be initiated.

Physiology and Pathophysiology (continued)

APH can occur from 20 weeks' gestation up to the onset of labor. IPH can occur between onset of labor and delivery. APH and IPH can be caused by the following:

- Abnormal placental attachment (eg, placenta previa, accreta, increta, and percreta)
- Uteroplacental separation (eg, placental abruption)
- Uterine rupture or trauma
- Fallopian tube rupture (eg, ectopic pregnancy)
- Fetoplacental vessel rupture (eg, vasa previa)
- Lower genital tract lesions (eg, cervicitis and vaginal varices)
- Spontaneous abortion

PPH can occur immediately after delivery and for up to 6 weeks after delivery. *PPH* is defined as a blood loss greater than 500 mL after vaginal delivery and greater than 1,000 mL after cesarean delivery. Uterine atony is a frequent cause of PPH and results from failure of endogenous maternal uterotonics (eg, oxytocin and prostaglandins) to stimulate effective contraction of the uterine musculature for adequate compression of the uterine blood vessels following delivery.

Other causes of PPH include the following:

1. Retained products of conception
2. Abnormal placental attachment
3. Uterine inversion
4. Coagulopathy
5. Gynecologic lacerations and tears
6. Uterine rupture

Signs and Symptoms

Respiratory
- Cyanosis
- Hypercarbia
- Hypoxia
- Pallor
- Respiratory arrest

Cardiovascular
- Cardiac arrest
- Delayed capillary refill
- Dysrhythmias
- Hypertension (early compensatory sign of hemorrhage)
- Hypotension (late sign associated with hemorrhage)
- Tachycardia

Neurologic
- Acute onset nausea and/or vomiting
- Altered or loss of consciousness

Renal
- Decreased urine output

Hematologic
- Abnormal laboratory study results:
  1. Altered coagulation study results
  2. Decreased hemoglobin and hematocrit values
- DIC
- Extreme observed blood loss
- Indications of DIC or coagulopathy (eg, oozing from puncture sites, uncontrolled bleeding, decreased fibrinogen levels)

Other Considerations
- Abdominal pain
- Estimated blood loss greater than 1,000 mL
- Fetal bradycardia or decelerations
- Vaginal or perineal bleeding

Differential Diagnosis

Obstetric Considerations
- Amniotic fluid embolism (see Chapter 17)
- Antepartum and intrapartum hemorrhage:
  1. Ectopic pregnancy
  2. Lower genital tract lesions (eg, cervicitis, vulvovaginal varices)
  3. Placental abruption
  4. Placenta previa
  5. Uterine rupture
  6. Vasa previa
- Postpartum hemorrhage:
  1. Placenta accreta, increta, or percreta
  2. Retained placenta
  3. Trauma to obstetric anatomy (eg, cervix, vagina)
  4. Uterine atony
  5. Uterine inversion
- Preeclampsia (see Chapter 32)
- Uterine trauma

Cardiovascular
- Aortocaval compression
- Hemorrhage (see Chapter 18)
- Hypotension (see Chapter 22)
- Hypovolemia

Renal
- Acute renal failure (see Chapter 33)

Hematologic
- Coagulopathy (eg, DIC, preeclampsia, anticoagulants, preexisting bleeding disorders, dilutional thrombocytopenia)

Other Considerations
- Hypocalcemia (see Chapter 16)
- Hypothermia (see Chapter 23)
- Shock (see Chapter 34)

Suggested Readings

Bose P, Regan F, Paterson-Brown S. Improving the accuracy of estimated blood loss at obstetric haemorrhage using clinical reconstructions. *BJOG*. 2006;113(8):919-924.

California Maternal Quality Care Collaborative. http://www.cmqcc. org. Accessed April 1, 2011.

Mayer DC, Smith KA. Antepartum and postpartum hemorrhage. In: Chestnut DH, Polley LS, Tsen LC, Wong CA, eds. *Chestnut's Obstetric Anesthesia: Principles and Practice.* 4th ed. Philadelphia, PA: Mosby Elsevier; 2009:811-836.

Chapter 30
Pacemaker and Automatic Implantable Cardioverter-Defibrillator

Treatment

Perioperative
- Continuously monitor cardiac rhythm, rate, and peripheral pulse.
- Temporary pacing, cardioversion, and defibrillation equipment should be immediately available with patches applied to patient.

Preoperative
- Determine type and function of CRMD.
- Determine patient's intrinsic cardiac rhythm and dependence on CRMD.
- Determine if EMI is likely for surgical procedure.
- Consider consultation with cardiologist or manufacturer of CRMD.

Intraoperative
- Advise surgeon to:
  1. Use bipolar electrocautery or ultrasonic (harmonic) scalpel.
  2. Use the minimal electrocautery current required to cut or coagulate.
  3. Use intermittent electrocautery for short duration, at least 6 inches away from CRMD.
  4. Place grounding pad near surgical site and as far away from CRMD as possible.

Treatment (continued)

- If EMI is likely, place magnet over CRMD to:
  1. Program pacing function to asynchronous mode.
  2. Disable rate-responsive function.
  3. Suspend antitachyarrhythmia function.
- Manage potential CRMD dysfunction due to EMI.
- For emergency pacing, cardioversion, or defibrillation:
  1. Terminate all sources of EMI.
  2. Remove magnet from CRMD to restore function.
  3. If function is not restored, institute current ACLS or PALS guidelines for temporary pacing, cardioversion, or defibrillation.
- Consider pharmacologic treatment as per ACLS and/or PALS guidelines if dysrhythmias occur.

Postoperative
- Consult with cardiologist or CRMD manufacturer to restore CRMD function.

Physiology and Pathophysiology

During the course of a normal cardiac cycle, the conduction pathways and structural components of the heart work in coordination. This synchrony is vital for blood oxygenation and stroke volume, which ultimately lead to adequate oxygen delivery to peripheral and central tissues. Cardiac dysrhythmias represent conduction and/or structural aberrancies of the cardiac cycle. Medical management of cardiac bradyarrhythmias, tachyarrhythmias, and heart failure may include the

Physiology and Pathophysiology (continued)

placement of a CRMD (eg, cardiac pacemaker or implantable cardioverter-defibrillator).

Safe and effective perioperative management of a CRMD is imperative to minimize adverse outcomes such as (1) device or lead tissue interface damage, (2) failure of device to pace or deliver shocks, (3) pacing or shock delivery when not indicated, and (4) alterations in pacing behavior or reset to backup pacing mode. EMI may be misinterpreted as intracardiac impulses by a CRMD, giving rise to abnormal behavior and potentially resulting in severe adverse outcomes. Potential sources of EMI include the following:

- Electrocautery
- Radiofrequency ablation
- Lithotripsy
- Magnetic resonance imaging
- Radiation therapy
- Electroconvulsive therapy

Signs and Symptoms

Respiratory
- Dyspnea
- Hypercarbia
- Hypoxemia
- Pulmonary edema
- Tachypnea

Cardiovascular
- Cardiac dysrhythmias
- Hypotension
- Left ventricular dysfunction

- Loss of central and/or peripheral pulses
- Myocardial infarction or ischemia
- Myocardial lead tissue damage
- Right- or left-sided heart failure

Neurologic
- Altered level of consciousness
- Ischemic stroke
- Syncope

Differential Diagnosis

Cardiovascular
- Conduction cardiac disease
  1. First-, second-, or third-degree AV nodal block
  2. Brugada syndrome
  3. Fascicular or bundle branch block
  4. Q-T interval prolongation
  5. Sinus bradycardia with hemodynamic compromise
  6. Sinus node dysfunction (eg, sick sinus syndrome)
  7. Supraventricular tachycardia
  8. Torsades de pointes
  9. Ventricular fibrillation
  10. Ventricular tachycardia
  11. WPW syndrome
- Structural cardiac disease
  1. Cardiomyopathy (concentric or eccentric)
  2. Cardiopulmonary disease (eg, COPD)
  3. Congenital cardiac disease
  4. Coronary artery disease
  5. Inflammatory disease (eg, pericarditis)
  6. Postcardiac surgical intervention
  7. Right- or left-sided heart failure
  8. Valvular cardiac disease

Suggested Readings

American Society of Anesthesiologists. Practice advisory for the perioperative management of patients with cardiac rhythm management devices: pacemakers and implantable cardioverter-defibrillators. *Anesthesiology.* 2011;114(2):247-261.

Atlee JL, Bernstein AD. Cardiac rhythm management devices (part I): indications, device selection, and function. *Anesthesiology.* 2001;95(5):1265-1280.

Atlee JL, Bernstein AD. Cardiac rhythm management devices (part II): perioperative management. *Anesthesiology.* 2001;95(6):1492-1506.

Chapter 31
Pneumothorax, Hemothorax, and Tension Pneumothorax

Treatment

- Administer 100% oxygen.
- Maintain airway patency (eg, endotracheal intubation if respiratory distress occurs).
- Perform needle decompression by inserting a large-bore IV needle at the second intercostal space, midclavicular line on the affected lung.
- Place a chest tube on the affected side.
- Obtain sample for ABG measurement.
- Obtain chest radiograph and chest CT scan.
- Use ventilation strategy for acute lung injury:
  - Use low volume to avoid volutrauma (6 mL/kg).
  - Adjust respiratory rate to maintain normocapnia.
  - Minimize peak airway pressures to avoid barotrauma (< 30 cm H_2O).
  - Use PEEP (5-10 cm H_2O).
- Obtain CBC count and coagulation studies.
- Monitor and treat anemia and hypovolemia in the event of hemothorax.
- Avoid nitrous oxide administration.
- Perform cardiac resuscitation per American Heart Association ACLS or PALS protocol as necessary.

Physiology and Pathophysiology

A pneumothorax is caused by air that becomes entrapped in the pleural space of the lung, leading to compression and respiratory distress. A pneumothorax can result from a disruption between the alveoli and pleural spaces, exposure of the pleural space to atmospheric air, or, on rare occasions, anaerobic gas-producing organisms. There are 4 possible causes of pneumothorax:

1. Trauma: blunt, penetrating trauma, and rib fracture
2. Spontaneous: weakened pulmonary parenchyma (eg, COPD)
3. Iatrogenic: complication of central-line placement, volutrauma, barotrauma, biotrauma, and atelectrauma
4. Infectious: tuberculosis or pleural effusion

A tension pneumothorax develops when tissue at the site of the injury acts as a one-way valve. During inspiration, air becomes entrapped in the pleural space and does not escape during expiration. The accumulation of air in the pleural space dramatically compresses the affected lung, prevents effective diaphragmatic contraction, and exerts pressure in the mediastinum and contralateral lung. The increased intrathoracic pressure compresses the heart, great vessels, and contralateral lung, leading to decreases in cardiac output and further respiratory distress. A tension pneumothorax is a medical emergency that requires prompt identification and treatment.

A hemothorax occurs as a result of blood accumulating in the pleural space. Trauma (eg, rib fracture), infection, or iatrogenic mechanisms cause vascular damage and rupture, resulting in hemorrhage into the pleural cavity. A hemopneumothorax is the combination of pneumothorax and hemothorax (eg, air and blood within the pleural space). This pathophysiological process may progress to tension hemopneumothorax resulting in compression of the mediastinum and subsequent cardiac and respiratory decompensation.

Signs and Symptoms

Respiratory
- Absent or decreased breath sounds on the affected side of the lung
- Altered $ETCO_2$ waveform (tension pneumothorax and decreased cardiac output)
- Cyanosis
- Dyspnea
- Hemoptysis (hemothorax)
- Hypoxemia: SpO_2 less than 90%, PaO_2 less than 60 mm Hg
- Increased $ETCO_2$ and $PaCO_2$
- Increased peak airway pressure
- Pallor
- Paradoxical respiration
- Possible contusion, bruising, abrasion, or laceration on affected side of the chest
- Radiographic translucency on the affected side of the chest

- Subcutaneous emphysema
- Tachypnea
- Tracheal deviation away from the affected side (tension pneumothorax) of the chest

Cardiovascular
- Cardiovascular collapse after initiation of positive pressure ventilation (tension pneumothorax)
- Chest pain
- Hypertension (early sign)
- Hypotension (late sign)
- Jugular venous distention (may be seen in tension pneumothorax)
- Narrowed pulse pressure
- Tachycardia

Neurologic
- Altered level of consciousness

Differential Diagnosis

Respiratory
- Atelectasis
- Bronchospasm
  (see Chapter 8)
- COPD
- Empyema
- Endobronchial intubation
- Hypoventilation
- Pneumonia

Cardiovascular
- Cardiac arrest
- Cardiac tamponade
  (see Chapter 10)

Musculoskeletal
- Costochondritis
- Intercostal muscle spasm
- Obesity or excessive chest tissue leading to inability to auscultate breath sounds
- Rib fracture

Other Considerations
- Anaphylaxis (see Chapter 5)
- Equipment malfunction (eg, pulse oximetry, mass spectrometry, see Chapter 6)

Suggested Readings

D'Angelo M. Blunt thoracic injuries. In: Elisha S, ed. *Case Studies in Nurse Anesthesia.* Sudbury, MA: Jones & Bartlett; 2011:181-188.

Leigh-Smith S, Harris T. Tension pneumothorax: time for a rethink? *Emerg Med J.* 2005;22(1):8-16.

Noppen M, De Keukeleire T. Pneumothorax. *Respiration.* 2008;76(2): 121-127.

Stafford RE, Linn J, Washington L. Incidence and management of occult hemothoraces. *Am J Surg.* 2006;192(6):722-726.

Chapter 32
Preeclampsia and Eclampsia

Treatment

- Definitive treatment is delivery of the fetus and placenta.
- Assess for potentially difficult airway.
- Maintain blood pressure control (systolic 140-155 mm Hg, diastolic 90-105 mm Hg):
  - Magnesium sulfate (IV loading dose of 4-6 g IV over 20-30 minutes) followed by infusion (1-2 g/h IV), which should continue for 24 hours postpartum (monitor for hypocalcemia)
  - β-blockers (eg, labetalol)
  - Calcium channel blockers (eg, nifedipine)
  - Vasodilators (eg, hydralazine, nitroglycerin, or nitroprusside)
  - Opioids
- Prevent and treat seizures:
  - Magnesium sulfate (normal range, 1.7-2.4 mg/dL; therapeutic range, 4-8 mg/dL)
  - Propofol
  - Benzodiazepine
- Maintain intravascular volume (crystalloid, colloid, blood products).
- Monitor urine output.
- Obtain laboratory testing:
  - CBC count, including platelet count.
  - Coagulation panel, including fibrinogen level
  - Liver function tests
  - Renal function tests, including urine protein level

Treatment (continued)

- Spinal or epidural anesthesia is preferred in the absence of coagulopathy.
- Use rapid-sequence induction if general anesthesia is necessary.
- Consider arterial and CVP monitoring for severe preeclampsia.
- Methylergonovine administration is contraindicated.

Physiology and Pathophysiology

Preeclampsia is a condition that occurs during pregnancy and affects most organ systems. It is the third leading cause of maternal mortality. The condition can progress to severe preeclampsia with extreme hypertension, which may result in coagulopathy, pulmonary edema, renal dysfunction, liver dysfunction, myocardial infarction, cerebral edema, seizures, and intracranial hemorrhage.

The pathogenesis leading to the development of preeclampsia is not completely understood. However, the disease is associated with endothelial damage leading to an imbalance between thromboxane and prostacyclin, which results in the following:

1. Platelet activation and consumption leading to thrombocytopenia
2. Increased renal glomerular permeability causing proteinuria
3. Decreased production of vascular vasodilating substances
4. Increased vascular permeability
5. Increased sensitivity to endogenous vasoconstrictors such as norepinephrine and angiotensin

Physiology and Pathophysiology (continued)

Risk factors for developing preeclampsia are numerous and include maternal obstetric factors, comorbid conditions (eg, underlying hypertension), genetics, lifestyle, and a history of preeclampsia. The progression of the disease is variable and may be severe when initially diagnosed. Without warning, preeclampsia may rapidly progress from mild to severe and finally to eclampsia. The onset of preeclampsia frequently occurs between 20 and 34 weeks of gestation, and it is associated with increased maternal and fetal morbidity.

Signs and Symptoms

Mild Preeclampsia
- Edema and/or weight gain
- Hypertension (systolic > 140 mm Hg or diastolic > 90 mm Hg)
- Intravascular fluid volume deficit
- Proteinuria (> 300 mg per 24 hours)

Severe Preeclampsia
- Cyanosis
- Epigastric and/or right upper quadrant pain
- HELLP syndrome
- Hypertension (systolic > 160-180 mm Hg or diastolic > 110 mm Hg)
- Intravascular fluid volume deficit
- Neurologic symptoms (eg, headache, vision disturbances, malaise)
- Oliguria (< 400 mL per 24 hours)
- Pulmonary edema
- Renal dysfunction
- Severe proteinuria (> 3 g per 24 hours)

Eclampsia
- New onset of tonic-clonic seizures

Other Considerations
- Fetal distress
- Headache
- Intrauterine growth retardation

Signs and Symptoms (continued)

Other Considerations
- Magnesium toxicity
  - 10-12 mg/dL (loss of deep tendon reflexes)
  - 15-20 mg/dL (respiratory arrest)
  - > 25 mg/dL (asystole)

- Nausea and vomiting
- Oligohydramnios
- Paresthesias
- Pharyngolaryngeal edema

Differential Diagnosis

Cardiovascular
- Gestational hypertension
- Hypertension (see Chapter 20)

Neurologic
- Increased intracranial pressure (eg, cerebral edema, intracranial mass)
- Intracranial aneurysm or hemorrhage
- Migraine headache
- Stroke
- Underlying seizure disorder

Renal
- Acute renal failure
- Nephrotic syndrome
- Renal dysfunction (see Chapter 33)

Endocrine
- Pheochromocytoma
- Thyroid storm

Hematologic
- Coagulopathy (see Chapter 14)
- DIC
- Hemolytic anemia
- Thrombocytopenia

Gastrointestinal
- Gallbladder disease
- Pancreatic disease

Pharmacologic
- Local anesthetic toxicity (eclampsia and seizures; see Chapter 26)
- Magnesium toxicity
- Sympathomimetic drug use (eg, cocaine, methamphetamine)

Suggested Readings

Nezat G. Cesarean section. In: Elisha S, ed. *Case Studies in Nurse Anesthesia.* Sudbury, MA: Jones & Bartlett; 2011:407-415.

Osborne LA. Obstetric anesthesia. In: Nagelhout JJ, Plaus KL, eds. *Nurse Anesthesia.* 4th ed. St Louis, MO: Saunders Elsevier; 2010: 1103-1146.

Polley LS. Hypertensive disorders. In: Chestnut DH, Polley LS, Tsen LC, Wong CA, eds. *Chestnut's Obstetric Anesthesia: Principles and Practice,* 4th ed. Philadelphia, PA: Mosby Elsevier;2009:975-1007.

Turner JA. Diagnosis and management of preeclampsia: an update. *Int J Womens Health.* 2010;2:327-337.

Chapter 33
Renal Dysfunction

Treatment

- Determine and treat the underlying cause of decreased renal function.
- Maintain adequate blood pressure and end organ perfusion:
  - Administer vasopressor(s), drug and dose based on the degree of hypotension and patient's condition.
  - Consider type and crossmatch for blood product administration.
  - Consider administering recombinant human erythropoietin or PRBC before surgery to treat anemia.
  - Consider administering platelets, FFP, cryoprecipitate, or desmopressin before surgery if bleeding time is increased.
- Avoid nephrotoxic drugs and IV dye:
  - NSAIDs
  - Aminoglycoside antibiotics
  - Radiographic contrast dye
  - Inhalation anesthetics (eg, sevoflurane)
- Review laboratory results and manage appropriately (eg, CBC count, coagulation studies, electrolyte levels, renal function, glucose and hemoglobin A_{1C} levels, urine creatinine clearance, urine protein level, and digoxin level).
- Establish adequate IV access for surgical procedure.

Treatment (continued)

- Consider invasive monitoring:
  - Arterial line placement and ABG monitoring
  - CVP monitoring
- Consult with nephrologist and cardiologist.

Acute Renal Failure
- Cause should be identified early and treatment initiated to maintain kidney function.
- Maintain blood pressure and adequate volume status:
  1. Crystalloids (avoid lactated Ringer's if hyperkalemia exists)
  2. Colloids
  3. PRBC if anemia is present
- Begin renal replacement therapy:
  1. Dialysis
  2. Peritoneal dialysis
  3. Hemofiltration
  4. Kidney transplantation
- Maintain urine output of greater than or equal to 0.5 mL/kg/h.
- Secure the airway in the event of respiratory distress.
- Avoid ACE inhibitors or angiotensin II receptor antagonists, which can decrease renal blood flow.
- N-acetylcysteine can be administered before contrast dye.

Treatment (continued)

Chronic Renal Failure
- Treatment is supportive, and patient status should be optimized before elective surgery.
- Continue antihypertensive therapy (ACE inhibitors and/or angiotensin receptor blockers, β-blockers, calcium channel blockers).
- Administer dialysis within 24 hours before surgery.
- Avoid fluid overload.
- Consider use of dialysis catheter if IV access is difficult (consult dialysis department for use).
- Pad extremities, which are prone to nerve injury and skin breakdown.
- Assess other comorbid conditions that are associated with chronic renal failure (eg, hypertension, diabetes).

Physiology and Pathophysiology

Renal dysfunction can be acute or chronic and varies in severity across the continuum until ESRD occurs. Decreases in urine creatinine clearance and increases in serum creatinine concentration reflect decreases in glomerular filtration rate. The deterioration in renal function alters the kidney's ability to excrete nitrogenous waste products and to maintain fluid and electrolyte homeostasis.

Physiology and Pathophysiology (continued)

ARF is defined as a sudden loss of kidney function that can occur over a period of hours, days, or weeks. If the causes of ARF are recognized and treated in a timely manner, they can be reversed. Those at highest risk for ARF are elderly people and patients with comorbidities (eg, hypertension, diabetes) and/or any baseline renal insufficiency. ARF occurs because of prerenal, intrarenal, or postrenal causes (see Table 33.1).

CKD can progress from renal insufficiency to CRF, also known as ESRD. CKD is a gradual and progressive loss of the ability of the kidney to excrete wastes, concentrate urine, and conserve electrolytes. Patients eventually require dialysis or renal transplantation. Increases in serum creatinine level, BUN level, bleeding times, and urinary albumin level, as well as hyperkalemia, hypocalcemia, and anemia, reflect severe decreases in kidney function and an alteration in glomerular filtration. Diabetes mellitus and chronic hypertension are the leading causes of CKD. Chronic hyperglycemia eventually leads to kidney dysfunction due to a thickening of the glomerular basement membrane, mesangial cell expansion, and glomerular sclerosis. Chronic systemic hypertension causes intrarenal hemodynamic changes such as glomerular hypertension, which in turn leads to glomerular hyperfiltration, permeability changes, and glomerulosclerosis. Medications used during anesthesia may have prolonged effects in patients with renal dysfunction because of decreased elimination.

Table 33.1. Pathophysiology and Etiology of Acute Renal Failure

	Pathophysiology	Etiology
Prerenal failure	Decreased renal blood flow	Acute hemorrhage leading to decreased renal blood flow Aortic cross-clamping/dissecting aorta Arteriosclerosis Congestive heart failure Decreased cardiac output Hypotension Hypovolemia Large third space loss (ascites, following burn) Renal artery stenosis or disease Shock states
Intrarenal failure	Direct damage to renal parenchyma	Acute glomerulonephritis Acute tubular necrosis (caused by ischemia, nephrotoxic medications, or radiographic contrast dye) Interstitial nephritis Preeclampsia Renal vascular, glomerular, or interstitial disease or injury Rhabdomyolysis/myoglobinuria
Postrenal failure	Decrease in forward flow of urine leading to hydronephrosis and an interruption in normal kidney function	Bladder tumors Catheter obstruction or kink Pelvic tumors Prostatic hypertrophy Renal calculi (kidney stones)

Signs and Symptoms

Respiratory
- Dyspnea
- Rales
- Tachypnea

Cardiovascular
- Angina
- CAD
- CHF

- Dysrhythmias from electrolyte and/or acid-base abnormalities (eg, hyperkalemia)
- Edema
- Hypertension
- Orthostatic hypotension
- Pericarditis
- Peripheral vascular disease
- Tachycardia

Signs and Symptoms (continued)

Neurologic
- Cerebral vascular disease
- Confusion
- Headache
- Lethargy
- Peripheral neuropathy
- Seizure

Hematologic
- Anemia
- Coagulopathy
- Epistaxis

Renal
- Anuria
- Decrease in urine creatinine clearance
- Increases in serum creatinine and BUN concentrations
- Oliguria
- Proteinuria

Gastrointestinal
- GI bleeding
- Nausea and/or vomiting
- Weight loss

Musculoskeletal
- Fatigue
- Myopathy
- Osteodystrophy and muscle cramps from hypocalcemia

Integumentary
- Bruising
- Pruritic excoriations
- Sallow "dull" pigmentation
- Uremic frost

Differential Diagnosis

Respiratory
- Pulmonary edema

Cardiovascular
- Atherosclerotic vascular disease
- CAD
- CHF
- Hypotension (see Chapter 22)
- Hypovolemia
- Pericarditis
- Peripheral vascular disease

Neurologic
- Cerebrovascular disease

Renal
- ARF conditions: (see Table 33.1)
  1. Prerenal (reduced blood flow to the kidney)
  2. Intrarenal (direct kidney tissue injury)
  3. Postrenal (urinary flow obstruction)
- Nephrotic syndrome
- Obstructed urinary catheter
- Prior renal dysfunction or existing renal problems

Hepatic
- Ascites
- Hepatic cirrhosis

Endocrine
- Hypoglycemia
- Increased antidiuretic hormone secretion as a result of pain or surgical stress

Hematologic
- Anemia
- Blood transfusion reaction
- Coagulopathy (see Chapter 14)

Musculoskeletal
- Rhabdomyolysis

Other Considerations
- Hyperkalemia
- Major operative procedures with large amounts of blood loss or decreased renal perfusion (eg, cardiopulmonary bypass, abdominal and/or thoracic aortic aneurysm repair)
- Multiorgan dysfunction syndrome
- Preeclampsia (see Chapter 32)
- Sepsis
- Trendelenburg position can cause anuria due to pooling of urine in the bladder.

Suggested Readings

Garwood S. Renal disease. In: Hines RL, Marschall KE, eds. *Stoelting's Anesthesia and Co-Existing Disease.* 5th ed. Philadelphia, PA: Churchill Livingstone; 2008:323-347.

Hilton R. Acute renal failure. *BMJ.* 2006;333(7572):786-790.

Ouellette SM. Renal anatomy, physiology, pathophysiology, and anesthesia management. In: Nagelhout JJ, Plaus KL, eds. *Nurse Anesthesia.* 4th ed. St Louis, MO: Saunders Elsevier; 2010:694-726.

Chapter 34
Shock States

- Administer 100% oxygen.
- Intubate the trachea and provide mechanical ventilation.
- Determine type(s) of shock and provide specific treatment.
- Administer IV fluids (crystalloids and/or colloids).
- Administer blood and blood products as necessary.
- Maintain appropriate blood pressure (MAP > 60 mm Hg).
  - Decrease anesthetic depth.
  - Administer vasopressors and/or positive inotropic medications.
- Provide warming measures.
- Insert at least 2 large-bore peripheral IV lines.
- Insert invasive lines (arterial line, central line).
- Consider IV scopolamine and/or ketamine for sedation if severe hypotension is present.
- Obtain ECG.
- Monitor CBC values, coagulation status, renal function, and electrolyte status, and manage appropriately.
- Monitor acid-base status.
- Monitor urine output (> 0.5 mL/kg/h).
- Perform cardiac resuscitation per American Heart Association ACLS and/or PALS protocol as necessary.

Physiology and Pathophysiology

Shock is defined as decreased peripheral perfusion resulting in inadequate cellular oxygenation. The causes of shock are divided into 4 categories:

1. Hypovolemic (most common)
2. Cardiogenic (ie, myocardial infarction)
3. Cardiac compressive (ie, cardiac tamponade)
4. Distributive (eg, septic, anaphylactic, and neurogenic).

As a result of prolonged and/or severe oxygen deprivation, the ability of cells to create energy in the form of ATP is diminished. Cellular acidosis ensues as free adenosine and pyruvic acid (by-product of anaerobic metabolism) is converted to lactic acid. Lysosomes degrade and secrete autodigestive enzymes that further inhibit cellular function. Inflammatory mediators such as leukotrienes, C-reactive protein, oxygen free radicals, and prostaglandins are liberated and further decrease physiological performance by causing cellular edema and destruction. As a result, normal autoregulatory organ function is compromised.

This pathological process occurs over a continuum and is divided into the 3 stages of shock: (1) compensatory, (2) progressive, and (3) irreversible. The more rapidly the shock state is treated, the greater the chance of patient survival. The specific shock states, signs and symptoms, and differential diagnosis are included in Table 34.1.

Table 34.1. Signs, Symptoms, and Treatment of Various Shock States

Cause	Signs and symptoms	Treatment
Hypovolemic shock		
Major vascular disruption with blood loss Excessive fluid loss (eg, vomiting, diarrhea) Inadequate fluid intake Major burns	Tachycardia Initial hypertension followed by hypotension Oliguria Cool, clammy skin Anxiety and/or confusion Decreased CVP	Identify cause, stop blood loss Replace volume Administer blood and blood products Vasopressor and inotropic support
Cardiogenic shock		
Damage to cardiac tissue causing pump dysfunction from ischemia, contusion, and drugs or toxins	Hypotension Decreased pulse pressure (< 25 mm Hg) Tachycardia Increased CVP/PCWP Tachypnea Pulmonary edema Oliguria Cool, clammy skin Anxiety and/or confusion	Inotropic and vasopressor support Aspirin therapy Obtain serum cardiac markers (CK-MB, troponin I and II), ECG Consider transesophageal echocardiogram, pulmonary artery catheter monitoring, intra-aortic balloon pump, thrombolytic therapy, cardiac stent placement, coronary artery bypass surgery
Cardiac compressive shock		
Tamponade Tension pneumothorax with mediastinal compression	Hypotension Tachycardia Tachypnea Anxiety and/or confusion Increased CVP/PCWP **Cardiac Tamponade** Beck triad (hypotension, JVD, muffled heart sounds) Decreased pulse pressure (< 25 mm Hg) Tachypnea **Tension Pneumothorax** Decreased breath sounds Unilateral breath sounds Tracheal deviation Cyanosis Tachypnea Respiratory compromise	Identify and correct cause Pericardiocentesis (cardiac tamponade) Needle decompression in affected lung (pneumothorax) Chest tube placement in affected lung (pneumothorax) Inotropic and vasopressive support

Abbreviations: CVP, central venous pressure; PRBC, packed red blood cells; FFP, fresh frozen plasma; CK-MB, creatine kinase, M and B subunits; ECG, electrocardiogram; PCWP, pulmonary capillary wedge pressure; JVD, jugular venous distention; DIC, disseminated intravascular coagulation; CSF, cerebrospinal fluid; CBC, complete blood cell; ABG, arterial blood gas; LFT, liver function test.

Table 34.1. Signs, Symptoms, and Treatment of Various Shock States (continued)

Cause	Signs and symptoms	Treatment
Septic shock		
Infection by a micro-organism causing a systemic inflammatory response Severe burns Bowel perforation Major trauma Indwelling devices (eg, urinary catheters, central lines) Intravenous drug use	Hyperpyrexia (fever) Tachycardia Hypotension Wide pulse pressure Decreased CVP Tachypnea Mental status changes Conjunctival petechiae Oliguria Liver dysfunction Coagulopathy DIC	Provide IV antibiotic therapy Provide volume, blood, and blood products Provide inotropic and vasopressor support Remove and culture indwelling devices Obtain urine, blood, and/or CSF cultures, CBC count, electrolyte panel, renal function and coagulation studies, D-dimer, ABG analysis, LFTs, and urinalysis
Neurogenic shock		
Central nervous system damage (brain and/or spinal cord)	Hypotension Decreased CVP Bradycardia Neurologic dysfunction (paresthesias, paralysis) Warm, dry skin Hypothermia	Provide adequate volume Provide inotropic and vasopressor support Atropine for bradycardia Treat hypothermia *Caution:* Administration of succinylcholine may cause hyperkalemia after 24 h of injury.
Anaphylactic shock		
Antigen-antibody reaction Blood transfusion reaction Delayed hypersensitivity reaction	Pruritus Urticaria Angioedema Tachycardia Hypotension Decreased CVP Tachypnea Respiratory compromise (stridor, wheezing, arrest)	Identify offending agent and discontinue use Provide adequate volume Provide inotropic and vasopressor support as needed Consider administration of epinephrine, corticosteroid, antihistamine (diphenhydramine)

Abbreviations: CVP, central venous pressure; PRBC, packed red blood cells; FFP, fresh frozen plasma; CK-MB, creatine kinase, M and B subunits; ECG, electrocardiogram; PCWP, pulmonary capillary wedge pressure; JVD, jugular venous distention; DIC, disseminated intravascular coagulation; CSF, cerebrospinal fluid; CBC, complete blood cell; ABG, arterial blood gas; LFT, liver function test.

Signs and Symptoms

Generic to all shock states; see Table 34.1 for specific signs and symptoms for various shock states.

Respiratory
- Hypercarbia
- Hypoxemia
- Respiratory distress or arrest

Cardiovascular
- Dysrhythmias

- Initial compensatory hypertension followed by hypotension
- Tachycardia

Other
- Acidosis
- Decreased urine output

Differential Diagnosis

Respiratory
- ARDS
- Increased PEEP
- TRALI (see Chapter 37)

Cardiovascular
- Cardiac dysrhythmias (see Chapter 9)
- Embolism (see Chapter 17)
- Myocardial ischemia and/or infarction (see Chapter 28)
- Pressure on major vascular structures (by surgeon)
- Superior vena cava syndrome
- Valvular stenosis or insufficiency

Neurologic
- Parasympathetic nervous system predominance (ie, total spinal anesthetic, see Chapter 36)
- Traumatic brain injury
- Vasovagal response

Hepatic
- Hepatic failure

Pharmacologic
- Excessive anesthetic drug administration
- Excessive β-blocking drug administration
- Excessive insulin administration
- Excessive vasodilator drug administration (eg, nitro-glycerin or nitroprusside)

Differential Diagnosis (continued)

Other Considerations
- Acute adrenal insufficiency (see Chapter 1)
- Burn injuries
- Embolism (see Chapter 17)
- Hypocalcemia (see Chapter 16)
- Hypoglycemia
- Infection
- Malignant hyperthermia (see Chapter 27)
- Pancreatitis
- Trauma
- Uterine-induced vena caval compression
- See Table 34.1 for information related to specific shock states.

Suggested Readings

Association of Anaesthetists of Great Britain and Ireland. Blood transfusion and the anaesthetist: management of massive haemorrhage. *Anaesthesia.* 2010;65(11):1153-1161.

Heiner JS. Penetrating traumatic injuries. In: Elisha S, ed. *Case Studies in Nurse Anesthesia.* Sudbury, MA: Jones & Bartlett; 2011:167-179.

Treggiari MM, Deem S. Critical care medicine. In: Barash PG, Cullen BF, Stoelting RK, Cahalan MK, Stock MC, eds. *Clinical Anesthesia.* 6th ed. Philadelphia, PA: Lippincott Williams & Wilkins; 2009:1444-1472.

Chapter 35
Stridor

Treatment

- Consult current ASA difficult airway algorithm for strategies to maintain airway patency (see Chapter 13).
- Provide supplemental humidified oxygen and increase F_{IO_2} as needed.
- Assess airway patency, quality of breathing, and hemodynamic stability.
- Consider CPAP in an adult patient.
- Secure IV access when patient's age and condition permit.
- Provide a calm, nonthreatening environment to reduce anxiety and agitation, which may further increase airway resistance and work of breathing.
- Obtain necessary diagnostic tests (lateral cervical or chest radiography) as patient's age and condition permit.
- Acute supraglottitis:
  - Provide antisialagogue.
  - Secure patient's airway (tracheal intubation or emergency tracheostomy).
  - Administer appropriate antibiotics as indicated.
  - For severe supraglottitis that compromises adequate breathing, induce anesthesia with maintenance of spontaneous respirations (ketamine, inhalation induction, or intravenous induction).
  - Extubate in OR only after confirmed resolution of supraglottitis (improved medical condition, direct visualization, and cuff-leak test).

Treatment (continued)

- Laryngotracheobronchitis (croup):
  - Provide aerosolized racemic epinephrine.
  - Administer corticosteroids (eg, dexamethasone).
  - Secure airway (tracheal intubation) with a smaller than normal endotracheal tube to minimize tracheal edema.
  - Use helium-oxygen mixture (eg, heliox).

Physiology and Pathophysiology

Stridor describes the high-pitched inspiratory and expiratory sound caused by turbulent airflow through a partially obstructed airway. Stridor may be mechanical (eg, subglottic edema) or pathological, and treatment should be aimed at alleviating the underlying cause. Stridor occurs in the adult and pediatric populations; however, pediatric patients are most vulnerable to complete airway obstruction owing to their immature respiratory system. Because of the narrow caliber of a pediatric patient's airway, inflammation greatly increases airway resistance, leading to rapidly occurring respiratory failure.

These 2 distinct pathological processes are associated with similar signs and symptoms, making diagnosis difficult. Acute supraglottitis involves inflammation and edema of anatomical structures above the vocal cords (eg, arytenoids, aryepiglottic folds, epiglottis). In contrast, laryngotracheobronchitis involves inflammation and edema of anatomical structures below (subglottic) the vocal cords (eg, trachea, bronchi).

Signs and Symptoms

Respiratory
- Cyanosis
- Desaturation
- High-pitched noise during inspiration and/or expiration
- Hypercarbia
- Hypoxia
- Increased PIP
- Respiratory arrest
- Substernal retractions
- Tachypnea
- Use of accessory muscles

Cardiovascular
- Bradycardia (late sign; however, may be the first sign in a young child)

- Cardiac arrest
- Hypertension (early sign)
- Hypotension (late sign)
- Tachycardia (early sign)

Neurologic
- Altered level of consciousness
- Anxiety

Other Considerations
- See Table 35.1 for a comparison of the signs and symptoms consistent with supraglottitis and laryngotracheobronchitis.

Differential Diagnosis

Respiratory
- Airway edema after upper or lower airway surgery
- Airway fire (see Chapter 3)
- Airway obstruction
- Bacterial tracheitis
- Bronchospasm
- Craniofacial and airway abnormalities
- Enlarged tonsils or adenoids
- Foreign body aspiration
- Functional laryngeal dyskinesia

- Laryngeal neoplasm (laryngeal papillomatosis)
- Laryngeal trauma (mechanical, chemical, thermal injury)
- Laryngospasm (see Chapter 25)
- Macroglossia
- Peritonsillar abscess
- Pharyngitis
- Postextubation stridor
- Prolonged tracheal intubation

Table 35.1. Comparison of Supraglottitis and Laryngotracheobron-chitis in Pediatric Patients

	Acute supraglottitis	**Laryngotracheobronchitis**
Airway obstruction	Supraglottic	Subglottic
Onset of symptoms	Rapid (within 24 h)	Gradual (over 24-72 h)
Pathological cause	Bacterial infection (*Haemophilus influenzae* type B)	Viral infection
Most common age group	2-6 y	6 mo–6 y
Lateral cervical/ chest radio-graph findings	Enlarged epiglottis (thumbprint sign)	Narrowing of subglottic area (pencil point or steeple sign)
Laboratory findings	Neutrophilia	Lymphocytosis
Stridor and respiratory phase	Inspiratory phase	Inspiratory and expiratory phases
Fever	High grade (often > 39°C)	Low grade (rarely > 39°C)
Symptoms	Respiratory distress Early signs: agitation, restless-ness, tachypnea, tachycardia, and suprasternal or subcostal retractions Late signs: lethargy, pallor, cyano-sis, sudden cessation of stridor (total airway obstruction), and hemodynamic collapse Dysphagia and drooling Characteristic posture of sitting up and leaning forward	"Barking" or "brassy" cough Rhinorrhea Respiratory distress manifesting with early or late signs

Differential Diagnosis (continued)

Respiratory
- Retained throat pack
- Retropharyngeal abscess
- Severe tonsillitis
- Spasmodic croup
- Squamous cell carcinoma of larynx, trachea, or esophagus
- Subglottic hemangioma
- Subglottic stenosis (eg, prolonged intubation, congenital malformation)
- Supraglottic and/or subglottic edema
- Tracheomalacia and/or laryngomalacia
- Vocal cord paralysis (eg, recurrent laryngeal nerve injury)

Cardiovascular
- Vasculitis

Endocrine
- Riedel thyroiditis
- Thyroid goiter

Hematologic
- Angioedema (see airway obstruction, Chapter 4)

Musculoskeletal
- Jeune syndrome
- Juvenile rheumatoid arthritis

Other Considerations
- Anaphylaxis (see Chapter 5)
- Infectious disease (eg, diphtheria)
- Ludwig angina

Suggested Readings

Clark GD, Stone JA. Anesthesia for ear, nose, throat, and maxillofacial surgery. In: Nagelhout JJ, Plaus KL, eds. *Nurse Anesthesia.* 4th ed. St Louis, MO: Saunders Elsevier; 2010:921-941.

Shah RK, Stocks C. Epiglottitis in the United States: national trends, variances, prognosis, and management. *Laryngoscope.* 2010;120(6):1256-1262.

Sobol SE, Zapata S. Epiglottitis and croup. *Otolaryngol Clin North Am.* 2008;41(3):551-566.

Chapter 36
Total Spinal Anesthetic

Treatment

- Treatment is supportive until the cerebral plasma concentrations of the local anesthetic decrease
- If patient is conscious, administer 100% oxygen and provide reassurance.
- If patient loses consciousness, mask ventilate with 100% oxygen.
- Secure airway with endotracheal intubation.
- Consider rapid-sequence induction (Use caution with induction agents in the presence of severe hypotension.)
- Assess and maintain appropriate blood pressure.
- Administer IV fluid bolus (10 - 20 mL/kg).
- Administer vasopressor(s) for hypotension (eg, ephedrine, epinephrine).
- Administer atropine for bradycardia.
- Treat seizures with benzodiazepine or propofol.
- Consider avoiding phenylephrine because it can exacerbate bradycardia.
- Consider vasopressin infusion in the presence of refractory hypotension.
- Administer atropine for profound bradycardia.
- Perform cardiac resuscitation per American Heart Association ACLS or PALS protocol as necessary.

Physiology and Pathophysiology

During neuraxial anesthetic administration, high concentrations of LA medications can rapidly diffuse into the brain and result in profound bradycardia, hypotension, loss of consciousness, cardiac and/or respiratory arrest, and death. Specific causes that induce total spinal anesthesia include the following:

- Subdural injection
- Use of a hypobaric solution for spinal anesthesia
- Excessive LA administration into the subarachnoid space during spinal anesthesia
- Excessive LA administration into the epidural space via epidural needle or catheter
- Inadvertent placement of an epidural needle or catheter into the subarachnoid space (eg, dural puncture), resulting in excessive concentrations of LA in the subarachnoid space
- Epidural catheter migration into the subarachnoid space, resulting in excessive concentrations of LA in the subarachnoid space
- A valsalva maneuver initiated by bearing down and holding a breath or by straining while attempting to change positions causes epidural vein engorgement, resulting in increased pressure on the subarachnoid space. This can lead to the cephalad spread of increased concentrations of local anesthesia into the brain.

The severity of the signs and symptoms is dependent on the dermatome level of motor blockade, sensory blockade, and sympathetic nerve fiber blockade. Severe hypotension can occur because of profound β-fiber preganglionic sympathetic nerve fiber blockade. Phrenic nerve function is transmitted from C3 through C5 and allows for stimulation of the diaphragm and breathing. Furthermore, the cardioaccelerator fibers that arise from T1 through T4 transmit efferent impulses to maintain the SNS input to the heart. Cephalad spread of LA that migrates in significant concentrations above these vertebral segments will result in apnea and profound bradycardia, respectively. Constant vigilance is vital after administering a spinal anesthetic and/or epidural anesthetic, because once a total spinal anesthetic has occurred, supportive treatment is imperative.

Signs and Symptoms

Respiratory
- Aphonia
- Difficulty breathing
- Respiratory arrest

Cardiovascular
- Bradycardia if spinal nerve block extends above T1 dermatome level
- Cardiac arrest
- Dysrhythmias
- Hypotension
- Tachycardia

Neurologic
- Altered level of consciousness or unconsciousness
- Anxiety
- Fixed and dilated pupils
- Nausea and/or vomiting
- Seizures

Other Considerations
- Inability to move upper extremities

Differential Diagnosis

Respiratory
- Hypoxia (see Chapter 24)

Cardiovascular
- Aortocaval compression
- Hypotension (see Chapter 22)
- Myocardial ischemia/infarction (see Chapter 28)

Neurologic
- Bezold-Jarisch reflex
- Cerebrovascular accident
- Seizures

Pharmacologic
- Local anesthetic toxicity (see Chapter 26)

Other Considerations
- Hypoglycemia
- Subarachnoid injection (eg, hypobaric solution or excessive volume)
- Subdural injection

Suggested Readings

Bernards CM. Epidural and spinal anesthesia. In: Barash PG, Cullen BF, Stoelting RK, Cahalan MK, Stock MC, eds. *Clinical Anesthesia.* 6th ed. Philadelphia, PA: Lippincott Williams & Wilkins; 2009:927-954.

Olson RL, Pelligrini JE, Movinsky BA. Regional anesthesia: spinal and epidural anesthesia. In: Nagelhout JJ, Plaus KL, eds. *Nurse Anesthesia.* 4th ed. St Louis, MO: Saunders Elsevier; 2010:1045-1076.

Tsui BC, Finucane BT. Managing adverse outcomes during regional anesthesia. In: Longnecker DE, Brown DL, Newman MF, Zapol WM, eds. *Anesthesiology.* New York, NY: McGraw-Hill; 2008:1053-1080.

Chapter 37
Transfusion-Related Acute Lung Injury

Treatment

- Stop blood product transfusion immediately.
- Mild to moderate TRALI:
  - Provide supplemental oxygen.
  - Administer noninvasive supportive ventilation (CPAP or BiPAP).
- Severe TRALI:
  - Use invasive supportive ventilation (intubation and mechanical ventilation).
  - Provide low-tidal volumes (6-8 mL/kg) and low plateau pressures (< 30 cm H_2O) for lung protection and prevention of pulmonary volutrauma and barotrauma.
  - Provide PEEP of 5 to 10 cm H_2O to promote alveolar recruitment and distention.
- Administer fluids to maintain adequate MAP greater than 60 mm Hg and urine output greater than or equal to 1 mL/kg/h.
- Provide supportive measures:
  - Invasive monitoring (arterial line, PCWP)
  - Central venous access
  - Vasopressor medication(s)
  - Inotropic medication(s)
- Report TRALI to blood bank and initiate institution-specific transfusion reaction protocol.

Physiology and Pathophysiology

TRALI has become the leading cause of transfusion-related morbidity and mortality. The development of TRALI is associated with the administration of all blood products; including whole blood, PRBC, FFP, platelet products, cryoprecipitate, IV immunoglobulin, and stem cell preparations. TRALI is characterized by (1) alveolar-capillary damage, (2) altered pulmonary capillary permeability, and (3) pulmonary edema. Treatment for TRALI is aimed at supporting the patient's cardiopulmonary function.

Two theories have been proposed regarding the exact mechanism of TRALI. The "immune-antibody" mechanism theory postulates that donor leukocyte antibodies bind to recipient neutrophils. Antibody-bound neutrophils are then sequestered within pulmonary capillaries. Subsequent activation of these neutrophils by donor leukocytes releases bioactive products, which results in endothelial damage, capillary leakage, and acute lung injury. In contrast, the "two-step" mechanism theory proposes that a physiological stressor (eg, surgery, sepsis, or massive trauma) causes pulmonary endothelial activation. Endothelial activation increases the reactivity of circulating neutrophils, which are then sequestered within pulmonary capillaries. The second step, subsequent transfusion of biologically active antibodies or lipids in donor blood products, activates the primed neutrophils, causing the release of cytokines and vasoactive substances that induce acute lung injury.

Signs and Symptoms

Respiratory
- Cough
- Cyanosis
- Dyspnea
- Hypoxemia

○ Clinical signs and symptoms of hypoxia
○ Pao_2 less than 60 mm Hg while breathing room air
○ Pao_2 to Fio_2 ratio greater than or equal to 300

Signs and Symptoms (continued)

Respiratory
- Hypoxemia
  - Spo_2 less than 90% while breathing room air
- Noncardiogenic pulmonary edema
  - Absence of clinical signs of cardiogenic pulmonary edema (fluid overload, jugular venous distention, or S3 gallop)
  - Absolute B-natriuretic peptide (BNP) level less than 100 pg/dL
  - Bilateral pulmonary infiltrates on chest radiograph
  - Diffuse pulmonary rales on ausculatory examination
  - Edema fluid protein to plasma protein ratio greater than or equal to 0.6
  - Frothy or exudative pulmonary secretions
  - Normal CVP
  - Normal left atrial pressure
  - Posttransfusion BNP to pretransfusion BNP ratio less than 1.5

- Pulmonary artery occlusive pressure less than 18 mm Hg
- Tachypnea

Cardiovascular
- Hypertension
- Hypotension
- Tachycardia

Hematologic
- Laboratory findings
  - Demonstration of HLA class I or class II
  - Hypocomplementemia
  - Leukopenia
  - Matching leukocyte antibody-antigen in the donor-recipient
  - Monocytopenia
  - Neutropenia

Other Considerations
- Acute onset (within 6 hours of transfusion)
- Fever
- No existing acute lung injury before transfusion
- No relationship to alternative risk factor for acute lung injury

Differential Diagnosis

Respiratory
- ARDS
- Aspiration (eg, gastric contents or near drowning)
- Inhalation injury (eg, thermal or caustic chemicals)
- Reexpansion pulmonary edema (eg, postthoracic surgery requiring 1-lung ventilation)

Cardiovascular
- Cardiogenic increased pulmonary capillary pressure
  - Acute or chronic valvular disease
  - Cardiac dysrhythmias
  - Cardiomyopathy
  - CHF
  - Constrictive pericarditis
  - Left-ventricular failure
  - Myocardial infarction or ischemia
  - Pericardial tamponade
- Noncardiogenic increased pulmonary capillary pressure
  - Circulatory volume overload (ie, fluid overload)
  - Negative-pressure pulmonary edema
  - Pulmonary embolism
- Reperfusion pulmonary edema (eg, postpulmonary thombectomy, transplantation, or cardiopulmonary bypass)
- Shock states (see Chapter 34)

Neurologic
- Neurogenic pulmonary edema

Hematologic
- DIC
- Hypoalbuminemia
- Immune-mediated reaction

Pharmacologic
- Illicit drug overdose

Other Considerations
- Eclampsia
- High-altitude pulmonary edema
- Immersion pulmonary edema
- Infectious disease
- Systemic inflammatory response syndrome (eg, sepsis)

Suggested Readings

Looney MR, Gropper MA, Matthay MA. Transfusion-related acute lung injury: a review. *Chest.* 2004;126(1):249-258.

Triulzi DJ. Transfusion-related acute lung injury: current concepts for the clinician. *Anesth Analg.* 2009;108(3):770-776.

Waters E, Nishinaga AK. Fluids, electrolytes, and blood component therapy. In: Nagelhout JJ, Plaus KL, eds. *Nurse Anesthesia.* 4th ed. St Louis, MO: Saunders Elsevier; 2010:401-419.

Chapter 38
TURP Syndrome

Treatment

- Stop the infusion of irrigating fluid into the bladder.
- Maintain airway patency, adequacy of breathing, and circulation.
- Administer high-flow oxygen by face mask.
- Limit IV fluid administration.
- Obtain blood sample (hemoglobin and hematocrit and electrolyte panel) to assess for anemia and hyponatremia.
- Administer loop diuretic (eg, furosemide).
- Consider administering 3% or 5% hypertonic saline IV (caution: may cause central pontine myelinolysis with rapid infusion).
- Redraw blood samples for electrolytes level every 20 minutes to assess resolving hyponatremia.
- Administer anticonvulsant to increase seizure threshold and/or inhibit seizure activity:
  - Benzodiazepine (midazolam)
  - Propofol (caution with administration if severe hypotension exists)
- Perform cardiac resuscitation per American Heart Association ACLS protocol as necessary.

Physiology and Pathophysiology

During specific endoscopic procedures such as TURP or hysteroscopy, fluid is instilled to provide bladder or uterine distention, irrigation, and improved surgical visualization. TURP syndrome occurs when an excessive volume of irrigating solution (sorbitol or glycine) is absorbed into the systemic circulation. The resulting intravascular hypervolemia causes circulatory overload and dilution of serum sodium and plasma proteins. These serum components diffuse out of the intravascular space and into the interstitial space. The relative hyponatremia can cause mild, moderate, or severe neurologic and cardiac dysfunction (Table 38.1). Because mild neurologic changes frequently occur first, some experts recommend spinal anesthesia so the anesthetist can monitor the patient's neurologic status.

Factors that influence the amount of irrigating fluid that is absorbed include the following:

- Duration of the surgical resection (ideally < 60 minutes)
- Hydrostatic pressure of the irrigating fluid (determined by the height of the fluid bags relative to the patient)
- Peripheral venous pressure
- Quantity of open venous sinuses

Treatment for hyponatremia caused by TURP syndrome includes decreasing the intravascular volume, which decreases the intravascular pressure gradient and promotes remobilization of serum sodium and plasma proteins into the vascular space.

Signs and Symptoms

- See Table 38.1.

Respiratory
- Cough
- Shortness of breath
- Wheezes, crackles, or rales on auscultation

Cardiovascular
- Cardiac arrest
- Dysrhythmias
- Hypertension
- Jugular vein distention
- Tachycardia

Table 38.1. Neurologic and Cardiac Manifestations Resulting From Dilutional Hyponatremia

Serum sodium (mEq/L)	Neurologic manifestations	Cardiac manifestations
120	Dizziness Headache Nausea	Hypotension Possible widening QRS complex
115	Vomiting Restlessness Confusion	Bradycardia Widening QRS complex Elevated ST segment Ventricular ectopy
110	Loss of consciousness Seizures Respiratory arrest	Ventricular tachycardia Ventricular fibrillation Asystole

Differential Diagnosis

Respiratory
- Acute pulmonary edema
- Hypoxia (see Chapter 24)

Cardiovascular
- CHF
- Hypervolemia
- Myocardial ischemia and/or infarction (see Chapter 28)

Neurologic
- Altered level of consciousness
- Increased intracranial pressure (cerebral edema, intracranial mass)
- Primary seizure disorder
- Transient ischemic attack and/or cerebrovascular accident

Renal
- Acute renal failure

Endocrine
- Hypoadrenalism
- Hypothyroidism
- Syndrome of inappropriate antidiuretic hormone secretion

Pharmacologic
- Local anesthetic toxicity (see Chapter 26)

Other Considerations
- Anemia
- Glycine toxicity (transient blindness, altered level of consciousness, myocardial depression)

Suggested Readings

Elisha S. Transurethral resection of the prostate. In: Elisha S, ed. *Case Studies in Nurse Anesthesia.* Sudbury, MA: Jones & Bartlett; 2011: 469-480.

Smith RD, Patel A. Transurethral resection of the prostate revisited and updated. *Curr Opin Urol.* 2011;21(1):36-41.

Stafford-Smith M, Shaw A, George R, Muir H. The renal system and anesthesia for urologic surgery. In: Barash PG, Cullen BF, Stoelting RK, Cahalan MK, Stock MC, eds. *Clinical Anesthesia.* 6th ed. Philadelphia, PA: Lippincott Williams & Wilkins; 2009:1346-1374.

Index

I-J

T